WORKBOOK FOR LANGUAGE SKILLS

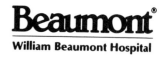

William Beaumont Hospital

*A complete listing of the books in this series
can be found online at wsupress.wayne.edu*

Series Editors
Michael I. Rolnick, Ph.D., CCC-SLP
William Beaumont Hospital

Alex Johnson, Ph.D., CCC-SLP
MGH Institute of Health Professions

WORKBOOK FOR LANGUAGE SKILLS

Exercises for Reading, Writing, and Retrieval

Second Edition
Revised and Updated

Susan Howell Brubaker, M.S., CCC-SLP

Wayne State University Press
Detroit

CONTENTS

6

RETRIEVAL

TARGET AREA 6: WORD RETRIEVAL

TARGET AREA 7: ANSWER KEY TO SELECTED EXERCISES

ABOUT THE AUTHOR

Susan Howell Brubaker has worked throughout her career in the Speech and Language Pathology Department at William Beaumont Hospital, Royal Oak, Michigan. For more than thirty years, she has specialized in working with adults who have suffered communicative loss as a result of neurological dysfunction or brain injury. She holds the B.S. from St. Lawrence University, Canton, New York, the M.S. from Ithaca College, Ithaca, New York, and the Certificate of Clinical Competence from the American Speech-Language-Hearing Association.

Other Susan Howell Brubaker books published by Wayne State University Press:

Sourcebook for Receptive and Expressive Language Functioning

Basic Level Workbook for Aphasia

Workbook for Aphasia:
Exercises for Expressive and Receptive Language Functioning
Third Edition (2006)

Workbook for Cognitive Skills:
Exercises for Thought Processing and Word Retrieval
Second Edition (2008)

Workbook for Reasoning Skills:
Exercises for Functional Reasoning and Reading Comprehension
Second Edition (2005)

INTRODUCTION

Communicative dysfunction related to neurological impairment is a significant rehabilitation problem in the educational and health care community. Adolescents and adults with language and cognitive disorders require specialized attention in order to achieve the highest potential possible. Specific clinical materials that address the identified level or levels of breakdown are critically important if effective help is to be given. Clinicians and teachers must search for those aids which will allow for appropriate and meaningful intervention.

—Michael I. Rolnick, Ph.D., Director, Speech and Language Pathology Department, William Beaumont Hospital, Royal Oak, Michigan

These words were written in 1984—exactly twenty-five years prior to the publication of the revised and updated second edition of this *Workbook for Language Skills*. Since then, thousands of copies of this workbook have been sold and many more thousands of pages have been used and/or given to adolescents and adults to aid in the process of their learning or recovery. In these intervening years, the field of speech and language pathology has developed and changed and grown in many ways; but one fact remains clear: relevant, appropriate, and quality treatment materials are still needed for individuals. While technological choices and evidence-based regimens are advancing—and rightly so—the use of paper and pencil for clear, uncomplicated independent work remains viable and even preferable in some circumstances. For this reason, in addition to its continuing popularity, the *Workbook for Language Skills* has been reborn after twenty-five years with a thorough makeover.

The makeover begins with the outside and continues on the inside pages of the book.

- A new tan ring binder, tabbed dividers with bold print, and sturdier paper keep the exercises fresh and easy to use.

- Newly formatted pages with larger, clearer print, visual line aids, and example boxes are designed to be user-friendly.

- The table of contents reflects clear divisions for the Reading, Writing, and Word Retrieval sections of the book with target area names that more clearly reflect their contents.

- Two exercises were omitted from the original version, and two new exercises were added.

- Extra pages have been added to twenty exercises.

- The questions in half of the book were rewritten, and vocabulary was changed to replace or update obsolete words or ideas, dated or politically incorrect references, and boring or repeated words or concepts.

- A user's guide has been added to give instructions, helpful suggestions and strategies.

- An assignments page has been added to help users keep track of what has to be done and to provide a useful record of progress over time.

- A totally new suggested answer key is included for most of the exercises.

We believe we have encompassed the best of the original book and hope that you agree that this revised and updated second edition is a much-improved tool that will help you the user or you the clinician achieve your goals.

Thank you for your continued support of Brubaker Books, your feedback, and your dedication to using our quality treatment materials to stimulate the brain and provide practice, a challenge, and perhaps even a chuckle or two.

Workbook for Language Skills targets those patients with moderate level expressive and receptive language deficits. It focuses on reading and word retrieval and has a secondary goal of spelling throughout the exercises. We use this workbook for our patients with both acquired and developmental communication disorders. Please use your clinical judgment to modify the tasks to meet your patient's needs. This revised edition will offer you more opportunities to work on language skills using terminology, situations, and names of people that are relevant today. As speech-language pathologists working in an outpatient rehabilitation facility, we have used this book in a number of ways over the years and are happy to share some of our ideas. A helpful addition is the new answer key located in Target Area 7.

We have listed some ideas and suggestions to maximize the usefulness of this workbook for speech-language pathologists and their patients:

- Use the table of contents as a way to identify a specific target area to focus on during treatment. Each section gives you multiple stimuli to address the target area in a variety of ways.

- Rather than explaining the directions for each task, allow patients to read the directions as a way to practice comprehension and retention skills through use of their strategies learned throughout their treatment program.

- As a functional way of improving auditory comprehension and retention skills, the speech-language pathologist can provide a verbal explanation of each exercise and then require the patient to restate the information.

- Use the examples to determine if the exercise is appropriate for your patient's level as this book has varying degrees of complexities in the target areas.

- Many exercises can address auditory comprehension. Rather than having the patient read the exercises, the clinician can present the stimuli auditorily.

- Many exercises can be modified to address verbal language from word retrieval to sentence formulation and beyond. Request a verbal response versus a written one.

- You can present an exercise in an open format to increase the response level. If your patient is unable to respond, you can offer the provided choices.

- When exercises are modified, the clinician has the ability to simplify and/or increase the complexity by altering the written choices.

- We often find that having patients note the start and completion time of an exercise helps them monitor their processing time. This helps with creating self-monitoring skills to manage impulsivity. It also shows the patient's improvement with speed of processing.

- Once an exercise has been completed, the speech-language pathologist can reassign the exercise at a later date to allow the patient to edit and elaborate on the original response using more complex and flexible thought processes. Providing the patient with the original response allows him to compare and celebrate his successes.

- Encourage your patients to compare their answers with the selected answer key located in the back of the book and to figure out why a mistake may have occurred. It should be taken into consideration that many items may have a number of reasonable answers.

- Give patients a personal copy of this workbook during their rehabilitation to enhance their ability to follow through with treatment tasks and compensatory strategies. We identify exercises that reinforce the goal addressed in treatment and assign these pages for completion prior to the next session.

- Assignments can be written on the assignments sheet in the front of the workbook. Strategies that are being worked on can be reinforced by listing them on the strategies page.

- Use of this workbook as a home program has additional benefits such as increasing self-direction, reinforcing a sense of accomplishment and confidence, and motivation for greater independence with communication skills.

- The inclusion of families and caregivers in home programming is paramount for a successful recovery. In our facility, families and caregivers take an active role in the rehabilitation process. They observe and participate in the use of this workbook facilitated by the speech-language pathologist and then are given workbook exercises to mirror the communication interactions in their home and social environments.

Susan Howell Brubaker has done it again! Her use of current language and vocabulary makes it easier to apply the target areas to the younger population as well as meet the needs of our adult population. As demands for cost-effective tools increase, this book offers clinicians treatment material that is wide-reaching, from the inpatient to the home care to the outpatient clinical setting. While the needs along the rehabilitation continuum vary, this workbook puts a variety of exercises at your fingertips. We look forward to incorporating this new book into our treatment regime.

Carolyn A. Doty, M.A, CCC-SLP
Manager, Outpatient Adult Services
Center for Adult Communication Disorders
Speech and Language Pathology Department

Lisa M. Mammoser, M.A., CCC-SLP
Coordinator, Diagnostics Program
Center for Adult Communication Disorders
Speech and Language Pathology Department

William Beaumont Hospital
Royal Oak, Michigan

STRATEGIES FOR THE USER

Make a list of things that will help you complete the exercises. This may include some strategies to help you do the exercise, recall words, spell words, or help you with the reading. Two strategies have been supplied for you.

1. First, read the <u>Directions</u>. If they don't make sense, read them again.

2. Look at the EXAMPLE. Read the question and the answer.

3. _____

4. _____

5. _____

6. _____

7. _____

8. _____

9. _____

10. _____

11. _____

12. _____

13. _____

ASSIGNMENTS

Refer to this page to remind you of what you have been assigned to do.

Date Assigned	Date Due	Pages

TARGET AREA 1:
Completions—Choices

TARGET AREA 1: Completions — Choices   Word Selection

DIRECTIONS: Each sentence has a blank. Choose one of the words below it that would best complete the sentence. Circle or write in that word.

EXAMPLE: The _____*train*_____ arrived at the station.

airplane   linen   order   (train)

---

1. The carpenter hammered the _____ into place.

    plant   nail   finger   bread

---

2. Trees usually lose their leaves in the _____ .

    rake   spring   fall   grass

---

3. The trash is picked up _____ Wednesday.

    on   in   of   with

---

4. There is _____ on tap.

    mayonnaise   beer   dirt   ammonia

---

5. I have run out of razor _____ .

    knives   shavers   blades   machines

---

6. I had a bowl of _____ for breakfast.

   toast   cereal   juice   eggs

---

7. The jewelry at _____ is expensive and of high quality.

   Kohl's   Panera   Tiffany's   Lowe's

---

8. You must _____ a room at the Hilton a week in advance.

   reserve   reverse   revere   repay

---

9. The dentist filled two _____ .

   cavities   seats   vases   jugs

---

10. The flashlight _____ was dead.

    flame   flash   electricity   battery

---

11. Jon gave a great acceptance _____ for his award.

    letter   meal   speech   present

---

12. There is a report of a _____ off the Gulf Coast.

    blizzard   contraband   fever   hurricane

13. The comedian told some _____ .

      jokes   plays   songs   dances

---

14. The curtains are being replaced with wood _____ .

      drapes   glass   blinds   shades

---

15. A lemon _____ pie just came out of the oven.

      juice   stew   soup   meringue

---

16. The winning candidate was sponsored by the _____ party.

      Surprise   Republican   Birthday   Dinner

---

17. She excused herself to put on fresh _____ after she finished her lunch.

      lipstick   deodorant   flowers   dessert

---

18. The printer has run out of _____ .

      paper   words   ribbon   wood

---

19. I'll have a glass of wine with my _____ .

      cereal   dinner   file   martini

20. Elton John performed many of his famous _____ .

    runs   products   hits   misses

---

21. The girl had lots of _____ on her face.

    freckles   polish   cheeks   hair

---

22. You need a good _____ to play tennis.

    glove   racket   goalpost   scalpel

---

23. Only one piece of chocolate _____ was left.

    grapefruit   candy   lettuce   milk

---

24. He picked up a _____ to read.

    tulip   shoe   magazine   chair

---

25. Did you buy anything at the _____ show?

    peep   art   talent   slide

---

26. The _____ on the pitcher is broken.

    lid   ceramic   chip   handle

TARGET AREA 1: Completions — Choices   Best Alternative

DIRECTIONS: Each sentence has a blank. Choose one of the words below it that best fits the sentence. Circle or write that word.

EXAMPLE: After it rained for two days, it was nice to see the

_____*sun*_____ come out.

moon   stars   (sun)   rainbow

---

1. The boxers were training hard for the _____.

   fight   race   game   trip

---

2. Baking bread _____ good.

   looks   feels   sounds   smells

---

3. The _____ belongs to the cat family.

   giraffe   tiger   anteater   catnip

---

4. I've seen _____ flying among the trees.

   cats   worms   twigs   robins

5. The _____ blew drifts as high as the window.

      tornado   blizzard   hurricane   thunderstorm

6. It was _____ so I put on a sweater.

      sold   dirty   Monday   chilly

7. You can go to Hertz or Avis to _____ a car.

      rent   sell   fix   wash

8. It's hard to know what to do with the pit of a _____ when you finish eating the rest.

      melon   peach   banana   raspberry

9. The animal with spots is the _____ .

      leopard   lion   antelope   raccoon

10. You must be _____ before you can vote.

      convicted   rewarded   registered   counted

11. I needed money so I _____ some from my bank account.

      stole   withdrew   deposited   saved

12. Original paintings can be a good investment because they may become

more _____ as they get older.

    moldy   faded   dusty   valuable

---

13. People often put chopped _____ eggs in their salads.

    scrambled   soft-boiled   hard-boiled   raw

---

14. The _____ on the pants broke.

    button   hem   zipper   jacket

---

15. Add a _____ of ketchup to the shopping list.

    carton   box   bottle   can

---

16. Vote for the _____ of your choice.

    nomination   candidate   position   election

---

17. Unless you wear your _____ your feet will
get soaked.

    umbrella   boots   hat   slippers

---

18. The car lights came on as I drove through the _____.

    bridge   airport   building   tunnel

19. A steady stream of _____ rose from the chimney.

   steam   smog   water   smoke

---

20. Lynn carried the _____ into the house.

   groceries   piano   leaves   skunk

---

21. Alex fell on the _____ and scraped his knee.

   snow   ball   mattress   gravel

---

22. Before he left on a road trip, he made sure his _____ was in good condition.

   jack   hubcap   piston   spare

---

23. It is already August; soon it will be _____ Day.

   Memorial   Valentine's   Independence   Labor

---

24. The _____ had the highest paying job in the company.

   receptionist   analyst   CEO   manager

---

25. You will need a _____ if you go camping.

   flashlight   lamp   TV   book

TARGET AREA 1: Completions — Choices   Most Sensible

DIRECTIONS: Read each sentence. Choose a word from the choices below the sentence that makes the best sense. Circle or write the word in the blank.

EXAMPLE: A _____*plumber*_____ fixes sinks.

teacher   (plumber)   mechanic   clerk

1. I'm going shopping; I need my _____.

   socks   umbrella   scarf   wallet

2. The three-year-old child was riding his _____ in the driveway.

   unicycle   tricycle   bicycle   motorcycle

3. There is no room for extra things, so you can only bring _____ items.

   essential   any   new   big

4. The restored Victorian home was honored by the _____ Society.

   Wilderness   Cancer   Humane   Historical

5. It has been raining so long there are

_____ warnings.

    tornado   flood   hurricane   storm

---

6. People could die of _____ during a famine.

    indigestion   starvation   measles   laryngitis

---

7. Putting good _____ in a home will help lower the heating bills.

    insurance   instrument   insulin   insulation

---

8. Someone who speaks from a pulpit to a congregation can be called

a _____ .

    builder   teacher   stockbroker   pastor

---

9. He brags a lot about his accomplishments; he is

very _____ .

    humble   egotistical   meek   open-minded

---

10. Block, tackle, and goalpost have to do with _____ .

    basketball   baseball   football   racketball

11. He was chosen from the audience to be a (an) _____ on the game show.

     emcee   sponsor   producer   contestant

---

12. Please send me a year's _____ to Newsweek.

     prescription   commission   subscription   permission

---

13. She sprained her _____ while she was jogging.

     neck   ankle   hand   shoulder

---

14. Trading on Wall Street is up; maybe it is a good time to buy some _____ .

     insurance   groceries   dividends   stock

---

15. If you are not a good swimmer, you should wear a life _____ in the canoe.

     jacket   boat   line   guard

---

16. Tourists often buy _____ to remind them of a trip.

     stamps   souvenirs   scissors   furs

17. A ball and a _____ are needed to play golf.

       mallet   club   paddle   bat

18. There are flowers on many graves in the _____ .

       nursery   cement   cemetery   garden

19. He measured the _____ of the door to see how long a piece of wood he would need.

       depth   color   width   height

20. Chocolate and butter are foods high in _____ .

       sugar   vitamin C   fat   iron

21. The judge will not take sides; he is _____ .

       partial   biased   neutral   stupid

22. If there is too much moisture in the air, you might buy a (an) _____ .

       humidifier   dryer   dehumidifier   air purifier

23. Installing a _____ alarm will warn you of a fire in your home.

       burglar   clock   false   smoke

24. The Olympics are an international competition

    in _____ .

    sports   spelling   debate   eating

---

25. The artist is painting a _____ of the twins.

    photograph   portrait   drawing   lesson

---

26. The lovely red _____ ring is worth $6,000.

    diamond   emerald   pearl   ruby

---

27. I have a _____ in my finger.

    splint   splice   splinter   spleen

---

28. I listen to the _____ on my ride to work.

    radio   birds   loudspeakers   television

---

29. My antique dining table is made of _____ .

    mahogany   bamboo   ivory   glass

---

30. A _____ is someone whose husband has died.

    bachelor   widow   widower   fiancé

TARGET AREA 1: Completions — Choices   Matching Facts

DIRECTIONS: Each word on the left has something in common with a word on the right.
Draw a line from the word on the left to the word it matches on the right.

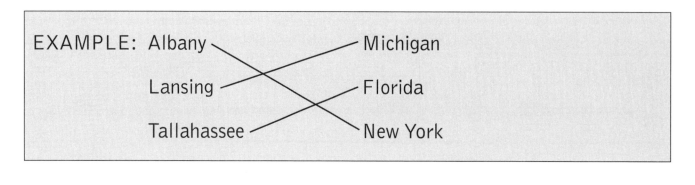

EXAMPLE: Albany   Michigan

Lansing   Florida

Tallahassee   New York

1. Rushmore   city

   Mississippi   mountain

   Seattle   river

   Pacific   ocean

2. Einstein   inventor

   Boone   Native American

   Geronimo   pioneer

   Edison   scientist

3. maple   blossoms

   oak   acorns

   evergreen   needles

   crabapple   sap

4. milk   carbonated

   cider   alcoholic

   soft drink   homogenized

   champagne   juice

5. Excedrin   detergent

   Windex   aspirin

   Tide   cleaner

   Mitchum   deodorant

6. Everglades   Pennsylvania

   Niagara Falls   Florida

   Golden Gate Bridge   New York

   Gettysburg   California

7. Ottawa   Japan

   London   India

   New Delhi   Canada

   Tokyo   England

8. Peter Pan   Gretel

   Prince Charming   Cinderella

   Red Riding Hood   Captain Hook

   Hansel   Big Bad Wolf

9. **60 Minutes**   movie

   Hamlet   TV show

   Star Wars   play

   Alice in Wonderland   book

10. Maya Angelou   composer

    Pablo Picasso   poet

    Mark Twain   artist

    Frederic Chopin   writer

11. Jamaica   continent

    Brazil   island

    Asia   country

    Geneva   city

12. Ronald   Bush

    George   Obama

    Barack   Clinton

    Bill   Reagan

13. sticks   piano

    keys   harp

    bow   drum

    strings   cello

14. colt   sheep

      kid   horse

      lamb   goat

      calf   cow

---

15. seeds   veins

      lead   pumpkin

      ink   pencil

      blood   pen

---

16. Michael Jordan   basketball

      Hank Aaron   football

      Walter Payton   baseball

      Wayne Gretsky   hockey

---

17. hamburger   omelet

      noodles   pizza

      dough   lasagna

      eggs   meatloaf

---

18. Tony Bennett   actor

      Jeff Foxworthy   politician

      Will Smith   comedian

      Rudy Giuliani   singer

TARGET AREA 1: Completions — Choices   Choices in Context

DIRECTIONS: Read the sentences, including the words in brackets. One of each pair of words in [brackets] does not fit. Cross out each word that does not fit.

EXAMPLE: **[Loafers ~~Beggars~~]** are a type of shoe. They **[~~do~~ do not]**

have shoelaces. They usually have **[low ~~high~~]** heels.

1. **[Restaurants   Theaters]** are places to eat. In a

    [sit-down   drive-thru] type, you choose food from a

    [menu   program] and order it from a **[dentist   server]**.

    Besides paying the **[bank   bill]** you usually leave a **[toothpick   tip]**.

2. An octopus has **[9 lives   8 arms]**. It lives in **[fresh   salt]** water.

    Some people like to **[eat   wear]** them. In some places, they are kept

    as **[decorations   pets]**.

3. **[Liberace   Shakespeare]** wrote many **[jokes   plays]**. One of

    his more famous is **[Macbeth   Oliver]**. He was from

    [England   Austria] and lived in the **[16th   20th]** century.

4. **[Benjamin   Herman]** Franklin started the nation's first

    [Starbucks   library]. He helped write the

    [Association   Declaration] of **[Independence   America]**.

    His **[home   picture]** is on the **[hundred   one]** dollar bill.

---

5. The **[treasurer   president]** lives in the **[Gingerbread   White]**

    House. He is the leader of the **[U.S.   U.N.]**. The nation's capital

    is **[New York City   Washington, D.C.]**. Two branches of

    [Supreme Court   Congress] are the **[Senate   Legislature]** and

    the House of **[Cards   Representatives]**.

---

6. A **[red   green]** light means to make a complete stop until the

    [red   green] light appears. You can often turn **[left   right]** after

    you make a complete **[U-turn   stop]** and you wait for any

    approaching **[police   traffic]** to clear.

Workbook for Language Skills copyright © Susan Howell Brubaker 2009

7. [Hummingbirds Cardinals] are the [most colorful smallest]

birds. They have [short long] bills that help them feed on

[seeds nectar]. Their [wings feet] make a humming sound as

they [fly sleep].

---

8. [Movies Books] are rated for the public. A [G X] rated movie is

recommended for any [age adult]. An [R X] rated movie is for

[children adults] only. A PG movie [is is not] appropriate for a

six-year-old to see.

---

9. [Raccoons Beavers] have broad [curly flat] tails. They have

[no buck] teeth to help them gnaw through [steel wood].

They can [swim fly] and build [dams bridges] across streams.

---

10. [Alaska Hawaii] is a [state country] made up of several

[islands continents]. It is located in the [Atlantic Pacific]

Ocean, and its capital is [Sacramento Honolulu]. A lot of

[pineapple tobacco] is grown there.

11. [Spaghetti Pizza] has a crust of dough usually covered with

[chocolate tomato] sauce, [cheese eggs], and other toppings.

It is [baked fried] and served by the [slice pound].

12. [Louis Neil] Armstrong is a famous [astronaut actor].

He commanded the [Apollo II USS Voyager] spacecraft that

landed on [Jupiter the moon]. He was the [only first] person to

[live walk] on the moon.

13. The [average oldest] person needs [4 7] hours of sleep a night.

Experts say that everyone [dreams snores] but not everyone

[remembers forgets] them. About [one-third three-fourths] of

people's lives are spent [dreaming sleeping].

14. A(n) [harp organ] is an instrument with many [locks keys].

You play the [locks keys] with your [hands feet] and the

[pedals strings] with your [feet hands].

TARGET AREA 1: Completions — Choices   Definitions

DIRECTIONS: *Each definition is incomplete. Put a check in front of the answer that best completes the definition.*

EXAMPLE: To go means to

_____ stop   ✔ leave

_____ hurry   _____ drive

---

1. To linger means to

   _____ run ahead   _____ lag behind

   _____ put away   _____ run away

---

2. To collapse means to

   _____ sit down   _____ roll up

   _____ fall down   _____ get up

---

3. Pastrami is a type of

   _____ pasta   _____ cheese

   _____ dessert   _____ meat

---

4. To unravel means to

_____ lift things   _____ plant things

_____ pull apart   _____ set aside

---

5. To anticipate means to

_____ look forward to   _____ handle carefully

_____ prevent   _____ look around

---

6. An antacid is

_____ an accomplishment   _____ a medication

_____ an injection   _____ a system

---

7. Flannel is a type of

_____ furniture   _____ fringe

_____ filter   _____ fabric

---

8. Vacant means

_____ empty   _____ unclean

_____ false   _____ delicate

9. Molasses is a

_____ place to hide   _____ dark syrup

_____ sticky surface   _____ soft drink

---

10. Whiskers are facial

_____ warts   _____ cosmetics

_____ hair   _____ blemishes

---

11. A document is

_____ a speech   _____ written information

_____ original   _____ confidential information

---

12. A spa is a

_____ family place   _____ religious retreat

_____ children's camp   _____ health resort

---

13. Incognito means someone is in

_____ pain   _____ disguise

_____ debt   _____ a box

14. A diagram is a

_____ muscle   _____ book

_____ picture   _____ disaster

---

15. To coax means to

_____ gently urge   _____ order something

_____ check over   _____ ask again

---

16. A virtue is something

_____ bad   _____ expensive

_____ good   _____ sour

---

17. To lounge means to

_____ sing   _____ exercise

_____ cook   _____ relax

---

18. To procrastinate means to

_____ delay   _____ eliminate

_____ enjoy   _____ finish

19. A decade is

_____ a card game   _____ an office supply

_____ ten years   _____ a child's toy

---

20. To terminate means to

_____ end   _____ listen

_____ goof   _____ pay

---

21. A sewer is a

_____ sponge   _____ machine

_____ drain   _____ metal stick

---

22. Cellophane is a

_____ cutting machine   _____ clear plastic

_____ carved candle   _____ case for a cello

---

23. A terrier is a

_____ delivery man   _____ material

_____ dog   _____ water

24. A bypass goes

     _____ on a trip   _____ around something

     _____ before a trip   _____ through something

---

25. A grenade is a

     _____ comb   _____ bomb

     _____ tomb   _____ womb

---

26. A dialect is a way of

     _____ listening   _____ acting

     _____ speaking   _____ writing

---

27. An option is a

     _____ nutrient   _____ direction

     _____ statement   _____ choice

---

28. A knuckle is a

     _____ finger joint   _____ toenail

     _____ head covering   _____ stomach cramp

Workbook for Language Skills copyright © Susan Howell Brubaker 2009

TARGET AREA 1: Completions — Choices   Multiple Answers

*DIRECTIONS: Each question has **six possible answers**. Put an **X** in front of <u>every</u> answer that could be correct. **HINT:** There may be more than one correct answer.*

EXAMPLE: What can you cook in an oven?

    _____ shoes   X casseroles

    X cake   _____ coffee

    X turkey   _____ ice cream

1. Where can you buy fresh fruit?

    _____ in an orchard   _____ in a restaurant

    _____ at a bank   _____ at a roadside stand

    _____ in a pool   _____ from a vending machine

2. What can you use to draw?

    _____ chalk   _____ a pencil

    _____ a joker   _____ a crayon

    _____ a marker   _____ a jar

3. What could fit in an envelope?

_____ a credit card   _____ a pillow

_____ a paper clip   _____ a basket

_____ a choir   _____ a snapshot

4. What do you keep in a refrigerator?

_____ cardboard   _____ soap

_____ sheets   _____ cheese

_____ cereal   _____ cream

5. What could you find in a library?

_____ palm tree   _____ books

_____ mayonnaise   _____ shelves

_____ movies   _____ maps

6. What would you keep in a linen closet?

_____ pillowcase   _____ shoes

_____ washcloth   _____ paint

_____ quilt   _____ cologne

7. What could you take for a headache?

_____ a bandage   _____ a warm drink

_____ an aspirin   _____ a haircut

_____ a nap   _____ a test

---

8. What do you eat with a fork?

_____ beans   _____ soup

_____ cake   _____ coffee

_____ ice cream   _____ salad

---

9. What can you buy at a drugstore?

_____ magazines   _____ shampoo

_____ gum   _____ comedy

_____ eggplant   _____ shoelaces

---

10. What can you put in a box you can carry?

_____ headphones   _____ a cabinet

_____ a pitcher   _____ a hernia

_____ a bathtub   _____ rags

11. What would you wear to keep warm?

    _____ a sleeveless top   _____ sandals

    _____ a sweater   _____ a wool jacket

    _____ shorts   _____ a bathing suit

---

12. What would be a good gift for a newborn baby?

    _____ a dictionary   _____ diapers

    _____ a teething ring   _____ a bib

    _____ a glass paperweight   _____ a stuffed animal

---

13. What would you keep in a safe-deposit box?

    _____ oranges   _____ a piano

    _____ deeds   _____ jewelry

    _____ stocks   _____ wills

---

14. What would you find in a greenhouse?

    _____ birdseed   _____ watering cans

    _____ luggage   _____ seedlings

    _____ dirt   _____ pots

15. What do you associate with computers?

_____ disco   _____ eBay

_____ Facebook   _____ Twinkies

_____ Gucci   _____ Google

---

16. What do you need to mail a letter?

_____ an envelope   _____ a stamp

_____ an address   _____ wrapping paper

_____ a box   _____ string

---

17. What do you need to play tennis?

_____ a court   _____ a racket

_____ an opponent   _____ a helmet

_____ cleats   _____ a net

---

18. What would happen at a traditional wedding reception?

_____ a toast   _____ a boat ride

_____ a food fight   _____ a tiered cake

_____ a garter toss   _____ a ring exchange

19. What should you save for income tax purposes?

    _____ past returns   _____ quarters

    _____ gum wrappers   _____ receipts

    _____ newspapers   _____ gas

20. What would you keep in a toolbox?

    _____ safety glasses   _____ a wrench

    _____ wire   _____ a blender

    _____ pliers   _____ a utility knife

21. What would you serve at a cocktail party?

    _____ ham and eggs   _____ cheese and crackers

    _____ chips and salsa   _____ steak and potatoes

    _____ ketchup and mustard   _____ popcorn and pretzels

22. What would you need on a camping trip?

    _____ candlesticks   _____ hairspray

    _____ an omelet   _____ matches

    _____ tent   _____ a lantern

TARGET AREA 1: Completions — Choices   Words in Paragraphs

DIRECTIONS: Each sentence has several blanks. Choose from the words below it to fill each blank. Each word is used once.

EXAMPLE: I drank a _____*cup*_____ of

_____*coffee*_____ before _____*dinner*_____ .

dinner   coffee   cup

1. Mr. Jones was selling his _____ . He put

   an _____ in the _____ .

   This _____ $12.00 a line.

   cost   paper   car   ad

2. We played _____ as we watched

   _____ . We also ate _____

   and drank _____ .

   TV   popcorn   poker   beer

3. There was an _____ at the

   _____ . The _____ had arrived,

   and an _____ was on the way.

   ambulance   intersection   police   accident

4. Because of the bad _____ the

_____ meeting was _____

for Thursday at _____ .

     8:00   weather   rescheduled   board

---

5. The sales _____ would not

_____ the _____ of

the _____ .

     refund   clerk   price   merchandise

---

6. There is a lot of _____ in

_____ . Some people believe this is

_____ to high _____ rates.

     movies   contributing   violence   crime

---

7. We are booked on a _____ to

_____ . Then we will

_____

by ship to _____ .

     travel   Miami   Nassau   flight

8. One _____ _____ cooked

_____ _____ , please.

    well   steak   medium   sirloin

9. _____ passed a _____

bill and _____ an energy bill during its

_____ today.

    Congress   vetoed   session   tax

10. Rush _____ _____

is _____ today for _____ .

    light   commuters   traffic   hour

11. _____ _____ show that

90% of all _____ own _____ .

    Americans   Government   statistics   cars

12. A good night's _____ , regular _____ ,

and multiple _____ help keep

one _____ .

    sleep   exercise   vitamins   healthy

13. The _____ restaurant has good

    _____ and the _____ one has

    great _____ .

        tacos   lasagna   Mexican   Italian

---

14. They spent all _____ in the

    _____ picking _____ so they

    could make _____ this afternoon.

        applesauce   morning   orchard   apples

---

15. College _____ is so _____

    that many people can't _____ to

    _____ it.

        high   afford   tuition   pay

---

16. The _____ had _____

    getting the baby to _____ for

    the _____ .

        pictures   trouble   photographer   pose

52

17. A _____ front is moving into the

_____ from the _____

bringing _____ _____ .

temperatures   state   west   cold   cooler

18. The _____ will give his annual

_____ of the _____

_____ on _____ .

Union   President   State   Wednesday   Address

19. Both Golden _____ and _____

make good _____ for _____

with _____ .

pets   Collies   Retrievers   children   families

20. A person who _____ _____

weather and _____ the _____

would enjoy living in _____ .

loves   cold   heat   hates   Florida

21. When he _____ how much the wall-mounted

_____ TV would _____ ,

he _____ that he could manage with a smaller

less _____ model.

    decided   cost   heard   expensive   plasma

---

22. Even though we set out a _____ , we can't seem

to _____ the _____ that

_____ under the _____ .

    lives   trap   raccoon   deck   catch

---

23. The _____ showed a small _____

in the _____ of the second _____

of my _____ .

    finger   fracture   X-ray   bone   joint

---

24. Two days after the _____ , our _____

was still out and _____ were _____

but some _____ were _____ .

    power   closed   schools   stores   storm   open

TARGET AREA 2:
Comprehension

TARGET AREA 2: Comprehension   Either / Or

DIRECTIONS: Answer each question by writing or circling one of the words from the question on the line.

EXAMPLE: Is a crocus a bird or a (plant)?

_____ *plant* _____

---

1. Is a smoothie a beverage or clothing?

   _____

2. Is **Family Feud** a game show or a soap opera?

   _____

3. Does a calculator use numbers or letters?

   _____

4. Is Columbus Day in the spring or in the fall?

   _____

5. Would a marine serve on land or water?

   _____

6. Is Tokyo the capital of China or Japan?

_____

7. Did Eve tempt Adam with a peach or an apple?

_____

8. Do people sing during a drama or an opera?

_____

9. Is a pendant worn on the neck or the wrist?

_____

10. Do you fuel a car with gas or oil?

_____

11. Do you eat a cantaloupe or a canteen?

_____

12. Do buffaloes live in the jungle or on the plains?

_____

13. If prices are inflated, are they higher or lower?

_____

14. In an assassination, is someone robbed or killed?

_____

15. Does an alcoholic drink or eat too much?

_____

16. Do you perspire more in hot or cold weather?

_____

17. Is it faster to jog or to crawl?

_____

18. Was Paul Newman a singer or an actor?

_____

19. Are moccasins for your feet or your hands?

_____

20. Would you tip a judge or a waitress?

_____

21. Is India a country or a continent?

_____

22. Could you watch a movie on an ATM or a DVD?

_____

23. Do you wear a helmet in football or tennis games?

_____

24. Is the tango a song or a dance?

_____

25. Is the Kentucky Derby a race for cars or horses?

_____

26. Would you count your steps with a pacemaker or a pedometer?

_____

27. Is tea made from beans or leaves?

_____

28. Is an autopsy ordered for someone who is alive or dead?

_____

29. Is pumpkin pie associated more with Halloween or Thanksgiving?

_____

30. Would a cut gemstone have facets or rivets?

_____

31. Is it more dangerous to be bitten by a rattlesnake or a garter snake?

_____

32. Would you clean up spilled milk with a broom or a sponge?

_____

33. If you were looking at a stage, would you be in an auditorium or a gymnasium?

_____

34. Do you need dice to play Scrabble or Yahtzee?

   _____

35. Would you find cuticles on your hands or your face?

   _____

36. Would you use a microwave or a microphone in the kitchen?

   _____

37. Is a praying mantis or a jack-in-the-pulpit a plant?

   _____

38. Do you need insulin or a tetanus shot if you step on a rusty nail?

   _____

39. If you wanted to get somewhere in a hurry, would you take a detour or an expressway?

   _____

40. Which is a tool: a trowel or a towel?

   _____

TARGET AREA 2: Comprehension   Facts

DIRECTIONS: Answer each question by writing **yes** *or* **no** *after it.*

EXAMPLE: Is Ontario in Canada? _____*yes*_____

---

1. Does a pentagon have five sides? _____

2. Does a ceiling fan run on batteries? _____

3. Is cinnamon a spice? _____

4. Is a lamb a young goat? _____

5. Can newspapers be delivered in the mail? _____

6. Can an elephant carry things in his trunk? _____

7. Do you eat yoga? _____

8. Do jellybeans grow on vines? _____

9. Is Listerine something to drink? _____

10. Can you squeeze a bowling ball? _____

11. Do pine trees lose their leaves in the fall? _____

12. Is Iran a country? _____

13. Do you record movies on a fax machine? _____

14. Will a vegetarian eat fruit? _____

15. Would you wear a cardigan? _____

16. Could you spend a sand dollar? _____

17. Are there 365 days in a leap year? _____

18. Is turkey a type of poultry? _____

19. Do you score a touchdown in soccer? _____

20. Has an American walked on the moon? _____

21. Do you serve yourself at a salad bar? _____

22. Can you wear suspenders? _____

23. Does a telescope make things look smaller? _____

24. Do people vote in a primary? _____

25. Is a tadpole a young frog? _____

26. Was Winston Churchill an American president? _____

27. Are basketballs and footballs filled with helium? _____

28. Do you cook an Eskimo Pie? _____

29. Is a koala something to drink? _____

30. Is Argentina in South America? _____

31. Does a cardiologist treat foot injuries? _____

32. Do you plant halogen bulbs in gardens? _____

33. Can you see through something transparent? _____

34. Is polio a sport? _____

35. Can you carry a cell phone in your pocket? _____

36. Do you need a prescription for aspirin? _____

37. Was Ebenezer Scrooge a senator? _____

38. Is the Mardi Gras held in Chicago? _____

39. Is Saturn a planet? _____

40. Was Buffalo Bill an animal? _____

41. Is Boston located on an ocean? _____

42. Do golf carts have handlebars? _____

43. Can you buy dandruff? _____

44. Does a conductor lead an orchestra? _____

45. Can you survive without your appendix? _____

46. Would you put chocolate sauce on an omelet? _____

47. Could you find a dormitory at a university? _____

48. Is being overweight good for your body? _____

49. Is a dead bolt a type of lock? _____

TARGET AREA 2: Comprehension   Abbreviations

DIRECTIONS: Each question contains some abbreviations. Answer each question by writing ***yes*** *or* ***no*** *after it.*

EXAMPLE: Are there 14 oz. in a lb.?   _____***no***_____

---

1. Does your Gov. live in Wash.?   _____

2. Do you have a 300 IQ?   _____

3. Does Wed. come before Tues.?   _____

4. Are there 52 wks. in a yr.?   _____

5. Is your wt. over 100 lbs.?   _____

6. Would you graduate from HS before a Univ.?   _____

7. Is LA in CA?   _____

8. Does your DDS fill cavities?   _____

9. Is Aug. the 6th mo.?   _____

10. Could a CPA help you with IRS forms?   _____

11. Is Mt. Rushmore in the USA? _____

12. Is FL NE of IA? _____

13. Does a man need to see an OB-GYN? _____

14. Is the legal speed limit 75 mph on a rd.? _____

15. Could you have cable TV in an apt.? _____

16. Is 17 an ex. of a no.? _____

17. Does the Pres. of the US have ESP? _____

18. Would you want an RN to treat you with TLC? _____

19. Can you get an MD degree before you get a BA? _____

20. Is NV on EST? _____

21. Is a dept. usually larger than a corp.? _____

22. Would a ¼ lb. burger be more filling than an 8 oz. steak? _____

23. Should you reply to an RSVP? _____

TARGET AREA 2: Comprehension   True / False

*DIRECTIONS: Each statement is either True (**T**) or False (**F**). Write **T** in front of the statement if it is true, and **F** in front of it if it is false.*

EXAMPLE: ___**T**___ The United States is in North America.

1. _____ Wolfgang Puck is a famous chef.

2. _____ A pelican is an Arctic bird.

3. _____ Raisins are made from dried grapes.

4. _____ Solar energy is powered by the sun.

5. _____ Wales is the capital of Scotland.

6. _____ Canada is ruled by England.

7. _____ Social Security is a type of burglar alarm.

8. _____ A plunger can be used to unclog a toilet.

9. _____ The Supreme Court is a singing group.

10. _____ Chili powder is a type of facial cosmetic.

70

11. _____ The Vietnam War was fought after World War II.

12. _____ Paris Hilton refers to a place in France.

13. _____ Rubik's Cube is a type of puzzle.

14. _____ ATM machines dispense food.

15. _____ Ravioli, fettucine, and gnocci are Italian pastas.

16. _____ Yosemite and Yellowstone are west of the Mississippi.

17. _____ Cocaine is a soft drink.

18. _____ Hybrid cars use hydrogen instead of gas.

19. _____ The tooth fairy brings teeth to people whose teeth have fallen out.

20. _____ Hostages are people who kidnap other people.

21. _____ Some pillows are filled with down.

22. _____ Bifocals and snorkels are both worn over the eyes.

23. _____ Studies show that smoking is linked to cancer.

24. _____   Velcro needs two different parts to work.

25. _____   A cardiac bypass refers to the kidneys.

26. _____   Cats use litterboxes more than people.

27. _____   ABC, CBS, and NBC are government agencies.

28. _____   A BLT sandwich stands for beef, lettuce, and tomato.

29. _____   A flute has strings.

30. _____   You could drink from a flask.

31. _____   Michael Jackson was a presidential candidate.

32. _____   Baseball games have innings and dugouts.

33. _____   Place mats and tablecloths are used for the same reason.

34. _____   An orphan can be adopted.

35. _____   A rabbit is a type of reptile.

36. _____   You might take an antibiotic if you have an infection.

37. _____ Rollerblades are special knives used to cut pizza.

38. _____ Some TVs will save a program so you can watch it at another time.

39. _____ E-mail stands for **elastic mail** because it can be stretched over long distances.

40. _____ Boston cream pie is really a cake.

41. _____ Lincoln Logs and Legos are used to build small models.

42. _____ The body's normal temperature is 98.6 degrees.

43. _____ Teddy bears can be dangerous to humans if they are protecting their young.

44. _____ Presidential elections occur every four years.

45. _____ You can buy merchandise through Amazon and ebay.

46. _____ New Orleans is also referred to as the **Big Apple.**

47. _____ Ben and Jerry are known for their many tasty barbecue sauces.

TARGET AREA 2: Comprehension

General Information

DIRECTIONS: Answer each question by writing **yes** *or* **no** *after it.*

EXAMPLE: Do you have fingernails on your feet? _____*no*_____

1. Would you call a dentist if you had heartburn? _____

2. Are pandas and penguins the same color? _____

3. Would you build a cabinet to live in? _____

4. Do you get salmonella from eating salmon? _____

5. Could you use a caddy in a golf game? _____

6. Do cars have steam engines? _____

7. Do you grow plants in a greenhouse? _____

8. Is an afghan usually found on a bed? _____

9. Can you boil water on the stove in a paper cup? _____

10. Do postage stamps have adhesive? _____

11. Does a digital clock have a second hand? _____

12. Do you buy shoes by the dozen? _____

13. Do giraffes have long ears and short necks? _____

14. Can you see a rerun more than once? _____

15. Is sign language used by the blind? _____

16. Would most people like to get a trophy? _____

17. Are Dutch people from the Netherlands? _____

18. Does American Express deliver packages overnight? _____

19. Is sushi something to eat? _____

20. Does dry ice keep things hot? _____

21. Do you usually learn to speak before you read? _____

22. Do men have abortions? _____

23. Do carbonated beverages have bubbles? _____

TARGET AREA 2: Comprehension   Reality vs. Fiction

DIRECTIONS: Read each phrase and decide whether it describes something that is possible or not. Put a plus (+) in front of something that could be real, and a minus (–) in front of something that could not be real.

EXAMPLE: ____ **—** ____ a striped giraffe

---

1. _____   a swollen ankle

2. _____   a phone that can take pictures

3. _____   a broken egg

4. _____   a 200-pound gopher

5. _____   a baseball team that wins all its games

6. _____   a flying carpet ride

7. _____   a seven-foot-tall person

8. _____   a clock that doesn't run

9. _____   a hen that lays golden eggs

10. _____   a wedding shower

11. _____ a haunted house

12. _____ a pen that corrects mistakes as you write

13. _____ a torn bathrobe

14. _____ a cat licking its horns

15. _____ a lost concert ticket

16. _____ a 10-year-old parrot

17. _____ shoes that grow as your feet grow

18. _____ a board with nails in it

19. _____ weathercasters who control the weather

20. _____ a bottomless jar of peanut butter

21. _____ a piano that plays by itself

22. _____ a case of sour grapes

23. _____ a spider with 10 legs

24. _____ a glass Ping-Pong ball

25. _____ a set of plastic dishes

26. _____ a truck that carries cars

27. _____ one pill that cures everything

28. _____ a light that turns off automatically

29. _____ a fireplace that does not use wood logs

30. _____ a kitchen that cleans itself

31. _____ bittersweet chocolate

32. _____ a dress with sequins

33. _____ a six-inch-tall hummingbird

34. _____ rusty water

35. _____ a 110-year-old woman

36. _____ a rainbow during a snowstorm

TARGET AREA 2: Comprehension   Desirable vs. Undesirable

DIRECTIONS: *This is a list of things that might happen to you. Some of them most people would enjoy, and some of them probably no one would enjoy. Put a plus (+) in front of something you would enjoy and a minus (–) in front of something you would* <u>*not*</u> *enjoy.*

EXAMPLE: <u> — </u>	be fired from a job
<u> + </u>	eat a good meal

1. _____   receive a compliment on your outfit

2. _____   be caught outside in a thunderstorm

3. _____   lose 15 pounds

4. _____   receive two free tickets to a show

5. _____   run out of gas on a country road

6. _____   live to be 105 years old

7. _____   slip on a patch of ice

8. _____   have a leak in your ceiling

9. _____   take a trip to Hawaii

10. _____ break a glass

11. _____ visit the White House

12. _____ be held hostage

13. _____ have your appendix removed

14. _____ buy something you really need at a big discount

15. _____ have a good night's sleep

16. _____ be bitten by a stray dog

17. _____ find an unexpected $20 in your wallet

18. _____ find a frightened skunk in your yard

19. _____ catch pneumonia

20. _____ have a massage

21. _____ receive a card from an old friend

22. _____ be in a car accident

23. _____   spill ketchup on your shirt

24. _____   go skydiving

25. _____   be a winning contestant on a game show

26. _____   see an animated film

27. _____   discover a large stain on your carpet

28. _____   make a delicious meal

29. _____   attend a party in your honor

30. _____   live next to a very noisy family

31. _____   go on a safari

32. _____   judge a cooking contest

33. _____   run out of hot water

34. _____   find a bug in your salad

35. _____   get very sunburned

TARGET AREA 2: Comprehension

DIRECTIONS: Read the sentence. Choose one or more words from the sentence to answer the question following it. Write this answer on the line or mark the answer words from the sentence.

EXAMPLE: The man was walking along the (side of the road.)

Where was he walking?   *the side of the road*

---

1. They went to Kroger to buy apple juice and paper towels.

   Where did they go shopping? _____

---

2. The photograph on the yellow wall was crooked.

   What was wrong with the photo? _____

---

3. Three of the five pencils on the table needed sharpening.

   How many pencils were on the table? _____

---

4. Hair grows faster on some people than on others.

   What grows faster on some people? _____

---

5. A mole can dig a 300-foot tunnel in one night.

   How long can the tunnel be? _____

6. I don't feel well, so I think I will sit down.

   What will you do? _____

---

7. She put soap and water on the tablecloth and rubbed hard to remove the spot.

   What was she using on the tablecloth? _____

---

8. He was so excited he ran up four flights of stairs.

   Why did he run up the stairs? _____

---

9. The current movie is about a handsome thief who smuggles valuable paintings.

   Who smuggles paintings? _____

---

10. The people who are picketing are yelling at the people who want to work.

    What are the people picketing doing? _____

---

11. The garbage pickup will be a day late this week because of the holiday.

    What will happen because of the holiday? _____

12. You must come to a complete stop before you can turn right on a red light.

   After you stop, what can you do at a red light? _____

---

13. The party was moved indoors when it started to rain.

   Why did the party go inside? _____

---

14. Most of the letters to the editor disagreed with the newspaper's point of view.

   To whom were the letters sent? _____

---

15. Insurance rates will increase 6 percent the first of the year.

   How much will insurance rates go up? _____

---

16. Each case contains 12 ten-ounce bottles of beer.

   How many bottles are in a case of beer? _____

---

17. The mattress costs $497.64 on sale and $649.95 regularly.

   How much does the mattress usually sell for? _____

---

18. Senior bowling is every Tuesday from 9 to 11 am.

   On what day do the seniors bowl? _____

19. Temperatures were in the 80s for three days in a row with humidity of 80 percent.

    For how long was the temperature in the 80s? _____

20. The heartbeat was loud and regular with a strong, even pulse.

    What was the pulse like? _____

21. We require two major credit cards and a driver's license before cashing your check.

    How many credit cards are required? _____

22. One tablet supplies all the body's minimum daily requirements of vitamins and minerals.

    How many minerals does a pill supply? _____

23. Herman's Deli will close on Thursday for remodeling.

    What's the name of the business? _____

24. The audience gave the actor a standing ovation.

    What did they give the actor? _____

25. He went on a strict protein diet because he wanted to lose 30 pounds.

    What kind of diet did he go on? _____

26. I keep my rings under lock and key.

   What do I keep out of sight? _____

27. The bank offers a $50 gift card if you open an account before the end of the month.

   What do you get if you open an account today? _____

28. We deliver orders over 20 dollars within a five-mile radius.

   Where do we deliver orders? _____

29. The high winds and fallen trees caused power failures in many areas.

   Where were the power failures? _____

30. Al from JMJ Roofing will come Monday before 12 to give an estimate.

   What is the company's name? _____

31. The brownie contains nuts and the cookie contains raisins.

   Which one has nuts? _____

32. We bought fresh doughnuts and candy apples at the cider mill.

   Did we buy cider? _____

TARGET AREA 2: Comprehension

Slang

DIRECTIONS: Each slang phrase has three possible definitions next to it. Mark the definition that is closest in meaning to the phrase.

EXAMPLE:

pep talk —— <u>an encouraging talk</u>

a talk about exercise

a religious talk

1. an only child

someone with no parents

someone with no brothers or sisters

someone with no relatives

2. a brainstorm

a fatal disease

an original idea

a type of weather

3. garage sale

a store for car parts

a way to get rid of a garage

a sale of things no longer needed

4. home plate

part of a baseball field

part of a set of dishes

part of a whole thing

---

5. coffee break

a game using sticks

a breakfast cereal

a time-out during the day

---

6. piggy bank

part of a pig farm

Miss Piggy's company

a place to keep money

---

7. car pool

a garage

a way of sharing rides

a swimming club

---

8. à la mode

with ice cream

in fashion

with mushrooms

---

9. empty nester

someone who is single

someone whose kids have left home

someone who has recently moved

10. hand-me-downs

a pair of hands

used clothing

a card game

---

11. graveyard shift

a job digging holes

a job in a cemetery

a job through the night

---

12. reality show

show with real people and situations

show that reviews new products

show with experts on childcare

---

13. box office

a company selling boxes

a place to eat

a place to buy tickets

---

14. cabin fever

allergies from an old building

distress from staying inside

illness in those who live in cabins

---

15. litterbug

someone who throws trash anywhere

a type of insect

someone who will eat anything

a type of weed

16. worrywart   a stressful skin condition

someone who worries a lot

---

an audition for actors

17. screen test   a spray for bugs and insects

a product for windows and doors

---

a specialty store for women

18. strip mall   an area with several connected stores

an area of government buildings

---

move a hen makes when laying an egg

19. chick flick   menu item that contains poultry

movie that females will probably like

---

bathrooms

20. restrooms   bedrooms

rooms with piped-in music

---

doctor's order for testing reflexes

21. gag order   judge's order to not talk about a case

teacher's order to stop talking in class

22. pack rat

someone who moves a lot

someone who saves a lot

someone who eats a lot

---

23. diva

woman who acts like a queen

man who dresses like a woman

woman who sings in operas

---

24. rain check

a weathercaster's tool

a place to hang umbrellas

a promise for the future

---

25. paparazzi

an Italian pasta dish

people who take celebrity pictures

a long hooded cloak

---

26. photo finish

very, very close first and second place

very beautiful scenery

a coating on a photograph

---

27. stay the course

to work overtime

to graduate before completing courses

to continue regardless of obstacles

TARGET AREA 2: Comprehension   Definitions

DIRECTIONS: Each definition has a choice of three words to fit it. Circle the word that best fits the definition.

> EXAMPLE: the distance from the bottom to the top
>
> area   width   (height)

1. it stops something from freezing

   defrost   antifreeze   unfrozen

2. to ship out of the country

   import   transport   export

3. a talk to learn about a person

   preview   review   interview

4. on the outside of something

   intramural   exterior   interior

5. to get rid of germs

   disinfect   infect   reinfect

6. loose coins

    exchange   change   interchange

___

7. not real

    artificial   factual   artistic

___

8. far away

    distinct   distant   discreet

___

9. turned down

    dejected   rejected   interjected

___

10. a group of cows

    herd   hoard   huddle

___

11. to remove the air from something

    dehydrate   inflate   deflate

___

12. ordinary and easy to find

    column   commence   common

13. very nice and enjoyable

    lovely   lonely   lowly

---

14. to get rid of errors

    connect   correct   collect

---

15. the person in charge

    worker   supervisor   visitor

---

16. anxious

    bored   nervous   proud

---

17. to see into the future

    predict   review   memorize

---

18. a fire that was deliberately set

    suicide   murder   arson

---

19. a legal way to bring a child into your family

    adoption   abortion   election

20. lightweight summer shoes

    slippers   loafers   sandals

---

21. a game using cards

    crossword   jigsaw   solitaire

---

22. someone who draws humorous situations

    balloonist   cartoonist   columnist

---

23. true to life; not made up

    fable   fiction   fact

---

24. having to do with the sun

    nuclear   polar   solar

---

25. to overstate the truth

    exasperate   exaggerate   exhilarate

---

26. a game with wickets and mallets

    croquet   polo   curling

27. recognition given for merit

    toward   award   reward

28. to cook with dry heat

    steam   boil   roast

29. to swallow large amounts

    gulp   gargle   sip

30. a dark coating on silver

    varnish   furnish   tarnish

31. not able to be read

    illegal   illegible   ineligible

32. a large company

    cooperation   corporation   corruption

33. to copy someone else

    imitate   intimate   imitate

TARGET AREA 2: Comprehension   Idioms

*DIRECTIONS: Read each sentence. Answer the question below it by marking **yes** or **no** after it.*

EXAMPLE: "You can't pin anything on me," said the suspect.

Should he be in jail?   yes   (no)

---

1. He cracked up when he heard the joke.

   Did he like the joke?   yes   no

---

2. I'm going to sow some wild oats before I get married.

   Is he going to be a farmer?   yes   no

---

3. The firm ended the year in the black.

   Was that a good thing?   yes   no

---

4. The surgeon has great skill but lacks in bedside manner.

   Is he warm and compassionate?   yes   no

---

5. They live on a cul-de-sac.

   Do they live on a dead-end street?   yes   no

6. He heard an ear-splitting noise.

   Was it loud?   yes   no

_____

7. The actors got three curtain calls.

   Did the audience enjoy the performance?   yes   no

_____

8. Our dishwasher has seen better days.

   Is it new?   yes   no

_____

9. They are going to tie the knot next week.

   Are they going sailing?   yes   no

_____

10. Trying to get the stain out of the rug was a lost cause.

    Was the stain hard to get out?   yes   no

_____

11. He slept with his security blanket.

    Was he a security guard?   yes   no

_____

12. He lost the race by a hair.

    Was he racing a rabbit?   yes   no

Workbook for Language Skills copyright © Susan Howell Brubaker 2009

13. I feel like a million dollars.

    Does he feel good?   yes   no

---

14. She is nuts about protein bars.

    Does she like them?   yes   no

---

15. He's like a bull in a china shop.

    Is he clumsy?   yes   no

---

16. She channel-surfed until she found what she wanted.

    Was she shopping?   yes   no

---

17. He drinks like a fish.

    Does he drink a lot?   yes   no

---

18. Her lips are sealed.

    Will she tell a secret?   yes   no

---

19. He's a pretty laid-back person.

    Does he get upset easily?   yes   no

20. That guy has some six-pack abs.

    Is he in good shape?   yes   no

---

21. She is going on a blind date.

    Is her date with a blind man?   yes   no

---

22. The generic brand of medication is now available.

    Is it probably cheaper?   yes   no

---

23. The Lions acquired the best draft pick.

    Are we talking about animals?   yes   no

---

24. Her boss docked her pay for being late.

    Was he glad she was late?   yes   no

---

25. The politician made an off-the-record remark to the reporter.

    Did he want his remark printed?   yes   no

---

26. He's fed up with all his junk mail.

    Does he like the mail?   yes   no

TARGET AREA 2: Comprehension   Same / Different

DIRECTIONS: Read the two sentences in each group. If the sentences mean the same thing,
write S for Same on the line in front of them. If they mean different things,
write D for Different on the line.

EXAMPLE: ___*S*___   He put on his right shoe last.

He put on his left shoe first.

---

1. _____   She slept until dinnertime.
She woke up. When it was time for dinner, she woke up.

---

2. _____   Everyone except Bob likes watermelon.
Bob likes watermelon.

---

3. _____   Throw the anchor overboard.
The anchor was over a board.

---

4. _____   The folded napkins were on the table.
Each of the tables had a folded napkin.

---

5. _____   The tomato plant was supported by the post.
The tomato plant couldn't stand by itself.

---

6. _____   She talks a lot.
She chatters constantly.

7. _____ Her leg had a black-and-blue mark.
There was a bruise on her leg.

8. _____ No one remembered to turn off the coffee machine.
The coffee machine was left on.

9. _____ Everyone except Mary liked the movie.
Mary liked the movie.

10. _____ The freezer was discounted 20 percent.
The freezer was on sale.

11. _____ The Johnsons never missed a game.
The Johnsons attended every game.

12. _____ Salmon is native to these waters.
There are no salmon in this stream.

13. _____ Be careful about what you eat.
Eat to your heart's content.

14. _____ Two men are in a blue boat.
Two blue men are in a boat.

15. _____ Smoking is strictly prohibited.
No smoking allowed.

16. _____ Wal-Mart is a chain store.

Wal-Mart is a store where you buy chains.

---

17. _____ She couldn't stand soap operas.

She was hooked on soap operas.

---

18. _____ Joe was convinced Jack should buy the cabin.

Jack convinced Joe to buy the cabin.

---

19. _____ The wind blew the paper.

The paper was blown by the breeze.

---

20. _____ The baker kneaded the dough.

The baker needed money.

---

21. _____ The movie got rave reviews.

The critics liked the movie.

---

22. _____ They ate lunch in no time.

They didn't have time to eat.

---

23. _____ The auditorium was crowded.

Many people were in the auditorium.

---

24. _____ Yesterday was Tuesday.

Today is Thursday.

25. _____ The soup was served before the salad.
    The salad was served after the soup.

26. _____ The passengers were boarding the jet at 2:15.
    The jet was ready to take off at 2:15.

27. _____ The red flowerpot was on the windowsill.
    The window had a red flowerpot on it.

28. _____ Some people prefer coffee to tea.
    Some people like tea better than coffee.

29. _____ Dogs can smell better than human beings.
    Humans have a better body odor than dogs.

30. _____ They are renting a car for the weekend.
    They are leasing a car this weekend.

31. _____ There's a reward being offered for the ring.
    A ring is being offered for the reward.

32. _____ He felt the paintings were judged fairly.
    The judges were painted at the fair.

33. _____ He bought an old piano for his wife.
    He bought his old wife a piano.

34. _____ He handled the situation with grace.
Grace had a handle on the situation.

35. _____ There are no better ribs than these.
These are the best ribs around.

36. _____ It took two years for Nick to save enough to go to London.
In two years Nick will go to London.

37. _____ We had chairs for 30 people, but 40 came.
Everyone had to stand.

38. _____ The clerk handed the woman her package.
The woman took her package from the clerk.

39. _____ He was pigeon-toed.
There was a pigeon on his toes.

40. _____ The light was dim in the restaurant.
It was hard to see in the restaurant.

41. _____ Kelly runs circles around Casey.
Casey is the fastest dog around.

42. _____ If I can't get it done today, I'll do it in the morning.
It will be done tomorrow at the latest.

TARGET AREA 2: Comprehension   Incongruities

*DIRECTIONS: Each sentence has a word in it that does not fit, so that the sentence does not make sense. Decide which word does **not** fit, and circle it.*

EXAMPLE: The box is too (light) for me to carry by myself.

---

1. We waited an hour at the station because the train was early.

2. The pool was drained, so I dove in for a swim.

3. The floor was swept with a vacuum.

4. I awoke to the chirping of the bees.

5. The chocolate had melted, so I put it in the oven to harden.

6. My feet were cold, so I put on some sandals.

7. The doctor said to take ten aspirin and go to bed.

8. The lightbulb burned out, so I changed the fuse.

9. Leave the roast in the freezer to keep it warm.

10. The aquarium had an exhibit of leopards.

11. The recipe for meatloaf called for ground beef and marshmallows.

12. There were flood warnings for the desert.

13. Eating cigarettes may be hazardous to your health.

14. The winning marathon runner was the last one to cross the finish line.

15. The Jacksons took their child to Subway for pizza.

16. The carpenter shopped for his tools at Hallmark.

17. The pitcher threw the ball to the quarterback.

18. You can always buy a good set of fingernails at a hardware store.

19. I walked up three flights in the elevator.

20. I get a yearly check-up at the doctor's every other month.

21. The mirror was so clean I could see my shadow in it.

22. They milked the cow and got chocolate milk from it.

23. My new green car runs on gas, electricity, and cola.

24. My butcher says a 14-ounce turkey will feed 20 people.

25. The NFL governs the rules of professional hockey.

26. The cat wanted to sleep somewhere soft, so it curled up on a board.

27. Most colleges offer choruses in a foreign language.

28. He hadn't slipped much during the night.

29. She is so strong she can hardly lift her purse.

30. She added a teaspoon of soap to the cookie dough.

31. No one in the back of the room could hear so his microscope was turned up.

32. When it gets really hot outside, I wear socks to bed.

33. Put the cake in the oven after you frost it.

34. Drinking a warm cup of iodine can soothe a sore throat.

35. Every fall the pine tree drops all its needles.

108

TARGET AREA 2: Comprehension   Inferential Questions

DIRECTIONS: Read both sentences. Then read the question under the sentences. Answer the question by marking the correct word below it.

EXAMPLE: Today is Tuesday
Yesterday was Monday.

What day is tomorrow?

Monday   (Wednesday)

1. The man is entering the store.
   The woman is leaving the store.

   Which one has finished shopping?

   the man   the woman

2. The cat is sleeping on a pile of dirty clothes.
   The dog is sleeping on the fireplace hearth.

   Which one is sleeping on something hard?

   the dog   the cat

3. They finished the chowder.
   They are eating the surf and turf.

   Have they had the cobbler?

   yes   no

4. The grass is turning green.
   You can see tiny buds on the trees.

   What season is it?

   spring   fall

---

5. Tom Hanks enjoys talking to his fans.
   Madonna does not like to be recognized in public.

   Who is more likely to give you an autograph?

   Tom Hanks   Madonna

---

6. The black squirrel chased the gray squirrel up the tree.
   The red squirrel was behind but gaining on them.

   Which squirrel was in the middle?

   red   gray   black

---

7. Harry is laid off from his steady job.
   Jane is working as a substitute teacher.

   Who is working this week?

   Harry   Jane

---

8. John won the race.
   Bob didn't finish the race.

   Who will not receive a prize?

   John   Bob

9. Most of my friends are taller and heavier than I am.

   Are my friends taller than I am?

   yes   no

---

10. Lucy has white paws and a long tail. She lives indoors and is declawed.

   What is Lucy?

   a cat   a dog

---

11. John wore a blue suit and white shirt and Bob wore blue jeans and a turtleneck sweater.

   Who was dressed casually?

   John   Bob

---

12. Four of us went to the movies and agreed the show was boring.

   Did we enjoy the movie?

   yes   no

---

13. During my week of vacation I flew to Niagara Falls, Manhattan, and Boston.

   Did I visit three states?

   yes   no

14. Rob put on his robe, ate his dinner, then took a nap.

    What did he do last?

    ate dinner   took a nap

---

15. The Smiths are going to the Johnsons to play cards Saturday.

    Who will be the hosts on Saturday?

    the Smiths   the Johnsons

---

16. My husband Harry's sister Mary is coming to visit.

    Who is coming to visit?

    Mary   Harry

---

17. He let the paint dry before he applied the shellac.

    What did he apply first?

    paint   shellac

---

18. Carol said, "Sam, did you get my message?"

    Who sent the message?

    Carol   Sam

19. Joan and Mark were married before she finished medical school and after he finished law school.

    Who had graduated when they got married?

    Joan   Mark

---

20. I slowly counted to 10, but then I lost my temper anyway.

    What did you do?

    counted to 10   lost my temper   both

---

21. She had driven 2 miles before she realized she had locked herself out of her house.

    Where were her keys?

    her purse   her car   her house

---

22. Harvey bought ice, cream, and cherries at the store.

    How many things did he buy?

    1   2   3

---

23. Mr. Riggs, a lawyer and financial analyst, will be here for dinner.

    How many are coming for dinner?

    1   2   3

24. Don asked Tim to send the proposal to John.

   Who will get the proposal?

   John   Don   Tim

---

25. Lisa, Bill's sister, is sitting next to Sue.

   How many people are sitting?

   1   2   3

---

26. The movie is shown at 10:00, 1:00, 4:00, and 7:00.

   How many afternoon showings are there?

   1   2   3

---

27. John is to the left of Jenny and to the right of Jane.

   Who is in the middle?

   Jane   Jenny   John

---

28. I heard a crack of thunder just after the lights went out and then I saw the lightning.

   What happened first?

   lightning   thunder   lights out

29. At the head table are: Pat the speaker who is next to Brad — an attorney with the company, Kelly who is CEO, and Pat's assistant.

How many people are at the table?

3   4   6

---

30. You can find do-it-yourself books in aisle 11, health books in aisle 4, and home decorating books in aisle 19.

If you want to fix your leaking toilet, which aisle should you go to?

4   11   19

---

31. Jay is wearing a sweatshirt. Todd is wearing a T-shirt. Nick has on a dress shirt.

Who is wearing short sleeves?

Jay   Todd   Nick

---

32. Before I read the front page, I look at the stock prices. I check the death notices before I look at the comics.

What do I look at first?

comics   stocks   headlines

---

33. Housing prices are off 20 percent, mortgage rates were just raised, and Ford's leasing rates dropped by 1.5 percent.

What is the good news?

housing   mortgage   leasing

TARGET AREA 2: Comprehension   Instructions

DIRECTIONS: Read the statements in each group. Then read the questions under the
statements. Write the answer to each question on the line.

EXAMPLE: Classical music is played on WRXZ at 101.5 FM all day.
Jazz is played on WXYP at 97.6 AM from 4–10.

When can you hear jazz?   *4-10*

What frequency is classical music played on?   *101.5*

---

1. Heat until boiling. Boil for five minutes. Lower the heat and simmer
   for 10 more minutes.

   What do you do for 10 minutes? _____

   Does it simmer before or after it boils? _____

   How long does it boil? _____

---

2. Lie on your back. Raise both legs slowly until they are about six
   inches off the ground. Slowly count to five, then lower your legs.

   Should you raise your legs together? _____

   For how long should you raise your legs? _____

   How far off the ground should your legs be? _____

3. Deal nine cards to each person. The person with the lowest diamond starts. If you can't discard, you must pick up a card.

What do you do if you can't discard? _____

_____

How many cards do you deal? _____

What suit starts the play? _____

4. Mix dry powder with equal parts of water. Use a wooden utensil to stir it. Scrape the sides of the can frequently. Stir at least three minutes.

Should you use a metal spoon to stir the paste? _____

How long should you stir it? _____

If you use one pint of paste, how much water should you use?

_____

5. Experienced salesperson wanted for work in jewelry store. Part-time position with flexible hours. Four years sales experience required. Prior work in jewelry design desirable.

Is this a 40-hour-a-week job? _____

Could an 18-year-old qualify? _____

What type of job is this ad for? _____

6. Before repainting a wall, scrape off any paint that has chipped or flaked. Then use sandpaper to smooth over the rough areas. If there are cracks or holes, use putty and a knife to fill them. Make sure the surface is even and clean before applying new paint.

Do you use putty after you paint? _____

What do you use to smooth the walls? _____

Should you paint over cracks? _____

7. Heat the oven to 425 degrees. Wash the potatoes with cold water and scrub off any extra dirt. Wrap the potatoes in foil. Put them in the oven and bake about an hour until they are done. To check for doneness, put a fork in one potato. If it is soft, it is ready to eat.

What do you wrap the potatoes in? _____

At what temperature do you bake them? _____

How can you tell if a potato is fully cooked? _____

8. Beverages or desserts should be served from the right. When plates are removed from the table, that should be done from the left. Put down utensils from either side.

From which side should a soup bowl be taken away? _____

Should coffee be served from the left? _____

Could you use your right hand to put down a butter knife?

_____

9. If you spill something on a carpet, you can often remove it with shaving cream. Squirt some of the shaving cream over the spot and rub it. Wash the spot out with water or club soda.

What can you use to clean some coffee that has spilled on a rug?

_____

Should you wash the spot with water before you use

shaving cream? _____

What do you do with the club soda? _____

_____

10. Cloudy tomorrow with a 60 percent chance of precipitation. Moderate winds picking up in the afternoon to about 30 miles per hour. High 68. Low 50. Humidity 40 percent.

What are the chances it will rain tomorrow? _____

What is the predicted low temperature? _____

How breezy could it get tomorrow? _____

11. Go up two flights of stairs. Turn left. Mr. Smith's office is Rm. 203.

Which way do you turn at the top of the stairs? _____

What room are you looking for? _____

What floor is the office on? _____

12. Turn left on Harris Street. Continue three blocks, then turn left at Vine Drive. Turn right at the first street onto Hill Road.

How many left turns do you make? _____

Do you come to Vine Drive before or after Hill Road? _____

How many corners do you pass on Harris Street? _____

13. Across from Henry Park, there are three houses. The middle house has two stories and is painted gray. The house to the left has red shutters and white trim. The house on the right is all brick, has lots of flowers in front, and is the largest house.

Is the brick house on the right? _____

Which house has white trim? _____

How many houses are described? _____

14. At the front desk, give Pat Fipps your name and tell her you have a 3:00 appointment with Jack Dunsburg. Ask for a registration form. Take it to a seat and fill it out. Be sure to use a blue pen and print the information.

What is the receptionist's name? _____

What should you use to fill out the form? _____

Who is the appointment with? _____

15. There is a showing at 8:00 and another one at 10:40. The box office opens at 6:45. Seating is first come, first served. Reservations must have been paid for prior to the evening of the performance.

    What time does the second showing start? _____

    Can you reserve a certain seat? _____

    Can you pay for your ticket the night of the performance?

    _____

16. The museum will be open on Saturday, March 9, from 10:30 to 3:30. Hours on March 10 will be from 1:00 to 4:00. Saturday's puppet show is at 11:00 for 45 minutes, and Sunday's candle-making demonstration is from 3:00 to 3:30.

    What are the hours on Sunday? _____

    How long does the demonstration last? _____

    If you want to visit the museum at noon, on what day would you

    have to go? _____

17. The house has been on the market at $269,900 for two months. It has 3 bedrooms, 2 baths, 3-car garage, and brick exterior. There is a dining area off the living room and a den that could be used as a bedroom.

    How many possible bedrooms are there? _____

    Is there a separate dining room? _____

    How long has the house been for sale? _____

18. Deodorant is in aisle 7 next to shampoo and below aspirin. Bandages are on the bottom shelf in the middle of aisle 9. Nail polish is in a separate display in the front of the store at the end of aisle 3.

    Is deodorant below shampoo? _____

    Is nail polish in aisle 7? _____

    What is in aisle 9? _____

19. The Investments course meets in room 101 from 7:30 to 10:00 Monday evenings. Art 101 meets Tuesday and Thursday from 8:00 to 10:00 in the cafeteria. Dog obedience is from 8:30 to 9:30 on Monday and Thursday in the gym. All classes run for six weeks.

    What time does course 101 meet? _____

    What meets in the gym? _____

    Which class meets for the most number of hours?

    _____

20. The recipe calls for the following ingredients:
    1 lb. fresh tomatoes or 1 12-oz. can of tomatoes
    1 lb. ground sirloin
    ⅔ cup chopped onions
    1 t. minced garlic (optional)
    ¼ cup cooking oil

    Do you use more oil or more onions? _____

    What can you omit? _____

    How much beef do you use? _____

21. The cream should only be used on a rash. Rub it on the affected area twice daily for ten days even if the rash disappears. If it gets worse, see a doctor. Do not take vitamin C pills while using the cream.

    Should you use the medicine every day? _____

    What ailment does the cream help? _____

    Can you drink a glass of orange juice while using it? _____

---

22. The **Grammy Awards** are on Thursday from 9 to 11 instead of **Ugly Betty** and **Grey's Anatomy**. One of the Batman movies and **Pretty Woman** are on cable at the same time. **Dancing with the Stars** can be seen just prior to the awards.

    When can you watch **Pretty Woman**? _____

    What is on at 8 o'clock? _____

    What would you watch at 9:00? _____

---

23. The pup is due for a shot in three months. She should be fed one cup of food three times a day until she is six months old. Check her nails weekly, brush her every other day, and give her a bath at least monthly.

    How often should she be brushed? _____

    What should happen in three months? _____

    How much food should the pup get daily? _____

24. I will have a Cobb salad with no bacon and extra cheese. I'd like
    Russian dressing unless it has onions in it. If it does, give me ranch
    dressing on the side. I want a baked potato with sour cream, no butter,
    and a side of parmesan cheese. And I'd like croutons on the salad.

    What extras go on the salad? _____

    What if there are onions in the dressing? _____

    What goes on the potato? _____

25. Kelly and Matt have registered at Macy's, Crate & Barrel, and Target.
    They have china but need glasses and silverware. They need sheets but
    have blankets. They want to pick out their own pillows. They picked
    out a coffeemaker and a food processor. They already have a blender.
    They need tablecloths and towels but no washcloths.

    How many things are listed on the register? _____

    What do they need to set a table? _____

    Do they have pillows? _____

    Do they need towels? _____

26. On Friday, Dan plays in a soccer game at 3 pm. Carrie has baseball
    practice from 10 to noon. Alex has golf lessons from 2:30 to 3:30.
    Dan's game is an hour away and the baseball field is a half-hour away
    in the opposite direction.

    What time should Carrie leave the house? _____

    Whose activities will overlap in time? _____

    Who will get the most exercise? _____

TARGET AREA 2: Comprehension

DIRECTIONS: There are three products, numbered 1–3, in each item. Below them are three instructions. Put the number of the product next to its instructions.

EXAMPLE: 1. plastic wrap   2. bandage   3. coffee

___2___   Remove backing, stick on area to be covered.

___1___   Pull to desired length, then tear off.

___3___   Add level teaspoon to cup of hot water.

1. aspirin   2. toilet cleaner   3. window cleaner

_____   Take two every four hours.

_____   Spray on, then wipe off.

_____   Remove labeling, put in position, and flush.

1. razor   2. rug cleaner   3. clock

_____   Spray with nozzle pointing down.

_____   Set time, set alarm.

_____   Carefully remove paper and slip in blade.

1. makeup   2. deodorant   3. shampoo

_____ Rub into hair, then rinse.

_____ Roll over entire underarm area.

_____ Dot lightly over face, then blend in.

---

1. peanut butter   2. salad dressing   3. can of Coke

_____ Shake before using.

_____ Lift and pull tab.

_____ Spread evenly on bread.

---

1. sweater   2. service counter   3. telephone

_____ Dry clean only.

_____ Press 0 to speak to a customer representative.

_____ Take a number and stand in line.

---

1. bank account   2. insurance policy   3. stock certificates

_____ Dividends will be paid quarterly.

_____ Your plan includes free checking.

_____ You have a $500 deductible.

126

1. library   2. cafeteria   3. doctor's office

_____ Please sign register and take a seat.

_____ Please dump trays when leaving.

_____ Book due on date stamped on card.

---

1. TV   2. radio   3. recorder

_____ Adjust control for FM.

_____ Adjust control for fast forward.

_____ Adjust control for vertical.

---

1. spaghetti   2. frozen juice   3. instant pudding

_____ Bring water to boil, add eight ounces, and cook.

_____ Add two cups milk to package and blend until thickened.

_____ Add three cans of water to concentrate and stir.

---

1. gas station   2. ice cream parlor   3. coffee house

_____ Choose no lead, regular, high octane, diesel.

_____ Choose single dip, pint, sugar cone.

_____ Choose espresso, latte, cappuccino, etc.

1. tea   2. cocoa   3. Kool-Aid

_____ Add one tablespoon to glass of water, add ice, and stir.

_____ Put two tablespoons in cup, add hot milk.

_____ Put bag in hot water and steep until the color you want.

---

1. fertilizer   2. wallpaper   3. nail polish

_____ Cut strip to one foot longer than needed.

_____ Sprinkle evenly over lawn.

_____ Spread evenly from cuticle out, then let dry.

---

1. rolls   2. frozen dinner   3. brownies

_____ Mix ingredients, spread batter in pan, and bake.

_____ Vent the cover and microwave according to directions.

_____ Pull dough apart and place on baking sheet.

---

1. cell phone   2. computer screen   3. microwave

_____ Push the time and power level before **Start**.

_____ Scroll down to view more information.

_____ Hit * for **Call Waiting**.

TARGET AREA 2: Comprehension   Expressions

DIRECTIONS: There are four slang expressions in each group with their meanings lettered from A–D. Write the letter of the meaning on the line that best describes the expression.

EXAMPLE: **_B_**   Take it easy.

         _A_   Beat it.

         A. Go away.
         B. Try to relax.

---

1. _____   I'm in the doghouse.

   _____   I'll grin and bear it.

   _____   I'm drawing a blank.

   _____   I'm on pins and needles.

   A. I can't remember.

   B. I'll put up with it.

   C. I'm very anxious.

   D. I'm in trouble.

2. _____ Snap out of it.

_____ Rise and shine.

_____ Knock it off.

_____ I had a change of heart.

   A. I reconsidered.

   B. Stop doing it.

   C. Change your attitude.

   D. Wake up.

---

3. _____ I'm all thumbs.

_____ I have a green thumb.

_____ I'm lightheaded.

_____ I lost my train of thought.

   A. I'm a good gardener.

   B. I'm feeling dizzy.

   C. What was I saying?

   D. I'm clumsy.

4. _____ It's a piece of cake.

_____ That rings a bell.

_____ It's a long shot.

_____ It's a matter of life and death.

    A. It's very important.

    B. It's very unlikely.

    C. It sounds familiar.

    D. It's very easy.

---

5. _____ Lend me a hand.

_____ Use your head.

_____ Keep a straight face.

_____ Start from scratch.

    A. Help me.

    B. Think about it.

    C. Begin at the beginning.

    D. Don't laugh.

6. _____ A stick-in-the-mud.

_____ A wolf in sheep's clothing.

_____ A pain in the neck.

_____ A jack-of-all-trades.

   A. An obnoxious person.

   B. An enemy posing as a friend.

   C. Someone who does not want to try new things.

   D. Someone who can do a little of everything.

---

7. _____ Megabucks

_____ Balderdash

_____ Shenanigans

_____ Diddly-squat

   A. Nonsense

   B. Nothing at all

   C. Mischief

   D. Lots of money

8. _____ She's in charge.

_____ She's having trouble making ends meet.

_____ Her lips are sealed.

_____ She's under the weather.

    A. She won't tell anyone.

    B. She doesn't have much money.

    C. She doesn't feel well.

    D. She is responsible for what happens.

---

9. _____ Chill out.

_____ Put a sock in it.

_____ Play it cool.

_____ Take a hike.

    A. Go away.

    B. Act confident.

    C. Calm down.

    D. Be quiet.

10. _____ Call it quits.

_____ Lose your cool.

_____ Throw in the towel.

_____ Break the ice.

    A. Stop what you're doing.

    B. Give up.

    C. Start talking.

    D. Get angry.

---

11. _____ Put in your two cents worth.

_____ Put your foot in your mouth.

_____ Put it on the back burner.

_____ Put the cart before the horse.

    A. Say something you regret.

    B. Do something later.

    C. Give your opinion.

    D. Do something in the wrong order.

TARGET AREA 2: Comprehension   Sayings

DIRECTIONS: Each statement has three possible meanings under it. Put a check in front of the saying that best describes the situation in the sentence.

EXAMPLE: He was depressed about the situation.

_____   He bit the dust.

___✓___   He was down in the dumps.

_____   He cried all the way to the bank.

---

1. I know it so well but I can't remember the name of the street.

_____   Forgive and forget.

_____   Business before pleasure.

_____   It's on the tip of my tongue.

---

2. I never thought I would miss him as much as I do.

_____   Misery loves company.

_____   Absence makes the heart grow fonder.

_____   Variety is the spice of life.

3. I really have to finish this work before I leave today.

_____ Never put off until tomorrow what you can do today.

_____ A spoonful of sugar makes the medicine go down.

_____ Things will work out for the best.

---

4. Don't give up; look everywhere you can think of.

_____ Two wrongs don't make a right.

_____ You win some, you lose some.

_____ Leave no stone unturned.

---

5. The weather is supposed to be sunny on Saturday, but just in case we will put up two tents.

_____ You're burning the candle at both ends.

_____ Hope for the best and prepare for the worst.

_____ Let a smile be your umbrella.

---

6. I can't believe you sold the coat I saw this morning. I came back to buy it.

_____ Get off my back.

_____ Here today, gone tomorrow.

_____ Life is what you make it.

7. That cheap toaster broke the first week I had it.

    _____ Take it or leave it.

    _____ You get what you pay for.

    _____ The end justifies the means.

---

8. Our group will never get anything done if all we do is argue about what to do.

    _____ Too many cooks spoil the broth.

    _____ You can't teach an old dog new tricks.

    _____ Every cloud has a silver lining.

---

9. There's nothing you can do about it now, so forget it.

    _____ All work and no play makes Jack a dull boy.

    _____ Don't beat around the bush.

    _____ Don't cry over spilled milk.

---

10. You sound just like your mother.

    _____ A chip off the old block.

    _____ A little frog in a big pond.

    _____ A lame duck.

11. You may say you're not still angry, but you're still frowning and yelling.

_____ You can't see the forest for the trees.

_____ Actions speak louder than words.

_____ You're a tough act to follow.

---

12. I knew I should have given myself more time to finish the project.

_____ Read between the lines.

_____ More bang for the buck.

_____ Haste makes waste.

---

13. Okay — I'll let you go to the mall if you'll just stop bugging me.

_____ Make up for lost time.

_____ The squeaky wheel gets the grease.

_____ Beggars can't be choosers.

---

14. He always sounds grumpy but he is a gentle soul with a heart of gold.

_____ An apple a day keeps the doctor away.

_____ You can't judge a book by its cover.

_____ All that glitters is not gold.

15. You are exactly right. We have been concentrating on statistics when we should have been improving our customer service.

    _____ You have your head in the clouds.

    _____ You hit the nail on the head.

    _____ You put the cart before the horse.

_____

16. It was supposed to be a surprise party for Gwen, but I guess Amy must have told Gwen about it.

    _____ Gwen got a dose of her own medicine.

    _____ Amy got the short end of the stick.

    _____ Amy let the cat out of the bag.

_____

17. This time let's toast to my old job and my new unemployment checks.

    _____ Start from scratch.

    _____ Drown your sorrows.

    _____ Keep your shirt on.

_____

18. This diet is so hard. I can't stand how little I can eat, and I am sick of salads.

    _____ Go jump in a lake.

    _____ Better late than never.

    _____ No pain, no gain.

TARGET AREA 2: Comprehension   Odd One Out

*DIRECTIONS: There are five items on each line. Four of them have something in common and one does not belong with the others. Cross out the item that does **not** belong.*

| EXAMPLE: eyelash | earlobe | ~~birthday~~ | armpit | cheekbone |

1. fiancée   vegetarian   snob   nephew   rodent

2. dominoes   computer   software   keyboard   CD

3. Pope   Vatican   Catholicism   priests   pyramids

4. tan   eggshell   cream   midnight   beige

5. chisel   wrench   pirate   file   pliers

6. cupcake   salad   tapioca   éclair   torte

7. mortgage   taxes   real estate   chains   foreclosure

8. linoleum   wallpaper   carpet   slate   hardwood

9. House   Den   Senate   Legislature   Court

10. marijuana   crack   cocaine   keys   pot

11. astronaut   space   satellite   launch pad   submarine

12. Captain America   Iron Man   Hulk   SpongeBob   Spider-Man

13. drums   rattle   clank   squeak   bang

14. PDA   ASAP   GPS   DVD   HDTV

15. bail   jail   crime   dime   parole

16. chili   sushi   alibi   salami   perogi

17. Titanic   Jaws   Gladiator   Psycho   Friends

18. stairs   press   news   media   reporters

19. firefly   briefly   butterfly   fruit fly   dragonfly

20. howdy	adios	ciao	sayonara	au revoir
21. picket	strike	foul	negotiate	contract
22. savings	interest	loans	deposit	accident
23. chandelier	heater	moon	candle	floodlight
24. quiche	benedict	omelet	au gratin	deviled
25. party	siesta	40 winks	nap	snooze
26. yarn	string	button	thread	twine
27. backpack	briefcase	tote bag	suitcase	closet
28. discount	rebate	bargain	markup	clearance
29. bachelor	aunt	groom	stepson	brother
30. cider	root beer	ginger ale	Sprite	Canada Dry

TARGET AREA 3:
Spelling

TARGET AREA 3: Spelling Word Recognition

*DIRECTIONS: There are three words on each line. Two of the words are spelled wrong.
One word is spelled right. Circle the **one** word that is spelled correctly.*

EXAMPLE: appel   opin   (box)

1. cource   buget   listen

2. fawset   onion   apeall

3. reelize   picture   orniment

4. motor   tungue   beleive

5. curtin   raindear   earning

6. speak   nuckle   girms

7. healthy   auktion   wellthy

8. remenber   commun   business

146

9. purposse	minite	sincere
10. journal	eegle	necesary
11. plastick	politics	piknic
12. normal	grosheries	ellectric
13. releif	awards	pronounse
14. unlimited	renewel	distanse
15. alligater	girafe	rooster
16. hyfen	organize	paintor
17. package	wiskers	ginjer
18. altarnate	detektive	leather
19. alarm	fether	hurrycane

20. crokus   bureau   divizion

21. alkahol   almunds   fabric

22. mineral   instument   dimond

23. romantick   lisence   performance

24. figure   lobstir   bearde

25. trophie   permenent   program

26. shingel   silence   carnaval

27. exibit   pertend   kidnap

28. thisle   warrent   manicure

29. frail   geraniem   dribbel

30. battiry   absorb   casuel

31. identical	exampel	underware
32. neighber	lokation	valuable
33. jealous	faverite	yestorday
34. bruther	kitchen	greasey
35. tomarrow	mattress	riverse
36. econamy	conquer	happyness
37. wrestling	parashute	liberary
38. humorus	sarcastick	dependable
39. yogort	recognize	nutritionel
40. boundry	misschief	diplomatic
41. exellent	ointment	important

TARGET AREA 3: Spelling   Alternative Spellings

DIRECTIONS: The same word is spelled three ways on each line. Two spellings are wrong and one is right. Circle the word with the <u>correct</u> spelling.

EXAMPLE:	ellelfunt	(elephant)	elephunt

1. fascility   fasillity   facility

2. champane   champagne   champaine

3. crocadial   crokedile   crocodile

4. dikshunery   dictionary   dictionery

5. vinyl   vinell   vinyel

6. acompanie   accommpany   accompany

7. absolutely   absulutely   absolutly

8. skying   skiing   skeeing

9. beautifull	beutiful	beautiful
10. suprize	sirprize	surprise
11. governor	governer	govorer
12. cumittee	comitee	committee
13. mayonase	mayonnaise	maionaise
14. vanila	vanilla	vannila
15. lunchun	luncheon	lunchin
16. pumpkin	pumkin	pummkin
17. sekretery	secratery	secretary
18. maxemum	maximum	maximam
19. ecsentric	eccentric	eccentrik

20. rackoon   raccoon   raccon

21. ordinary   ordeanary   ordinery

22. nusense   nuisance   nusance

23. fascinating   fasinating   fastenating

24. cedir   cedar   sedar

25. mekanik   mackanic   mechanic

26. memmorial   memorial   mamorial

27. guarantee   gerantee   garentee

28. plesure   plezure   pleasure

29. manipulate   munipulate   manepulate

30. territery   territory   tearatory

31. ocasion	occasion	occation
32. riythem	rythim	rhythm
33. November	Nouvember	Novembir
34. Februery	February	Febuary
35. miniachure	minature	miniature
36. volunteer	voluntier	volluntere
37. showlders	sholders	shoulders
38. rehearsal	rehearsil	reahersal
39. addaquit	adequate	adaquite
40. physitian	physician	phyission
41. abrrevation	abreviatian	abbreviation

TARGET AREA 3: Spelling   Accurate Spelling

DIRECTIONS: *There are three words on each line. Two of the words are spelled correctly.*
One word is spelled wrong. Circle the one word with the __incorrect__ spelling.

EXAMPLE: orange   addition   (carpit)

1. course   coopon   corner

2. hiccups   hungery   hobby

3. rooster   referance   residence

4. lowering   lengthen   lodgical

5. associate   anniversary   anounce

6. dignosis   dramatic   daughter

7. waffles   watermellon   wreath

8. language   laringitis   laundry

9. enamel	energetic	endevear
10. president	probabely	permission
11. spatula	spinatch	species
12. bicicle	bouquet	beneath
13. gorilla	groutchy	groceries
14. realistic	raisin	razsberry
15. innosent	immediate	imagine
16. niece	natuerally	nectarine
17. geranium	generous	gardner
18. umanimous	universe	unfamiliar
19. knowledge	karesene	khaki

20. technical	treasure	trajedy
21. jellousy	journalist	jewelry
22. marshmallow	medisine	memorize
23. valueble	variety	vegetable
24. fertilizer	fascinated	frushtrated
25. orchestra	orijinal	outrageous
26. hockey	holliday	horizontal
27. negoshiate	natural	navigate
28. wonderful	weapen	windshield
29. sandwich	scissors	sckedule
30. ellevater	essential	emergency

31. coconut	clearance	chockolate
32. reasonble	realize	receiver
33. leisure	laufhter	lavender
34. garage	gesture	generus
35. magician	mashine	macaroni
36. teaspoon	terrific	toester
37. delishious	democracy	decision
38. biology	blueberries	brillant
39. nowhere	nomminate	nightmare
40. opinon	octopus	objection
41. yawning	yoreself	yardstick

TARGET AREA 3: Spelling   Words from Blends

DIRECTIONS: Three letter groups are shown in the box. Add one of the letter groups to each blank to form a word. They can be used more than once.

EXAMPLE:	**or**	**ir**	**ar**

st _ir_____   e _ar____ th   _or____ gan

1.

sh	**ch**	**th**

_____ ort   _____ air   _____ est   _____ ere

_____ art   _____ en   _____ irsty   _____ ade

2.

ie	**ee**	**ei**

m _____ t   squ _____ ze   bel _____ ve   b _____ ng

p _____ ce   w _____ ght   c _____ ling   fr _____ nd

3.

be	**con**	**in**

_____ tain   _____ auty   _____ sult   _____ demn

_____ tinue   _____ dex   _____ fore   _____ lief

4.

ex	**un**	**per**

_____ tra   _____ ite   _____ act   _____ cuse

_____ cent   _____ haps   _____ happy   _____ form

5.

inter	trans	com

_____ mon   _____ port   _____ nal   _____ fer

_____ late   _____ plex   _____ view   _____ pany

6.

oo	ee	oa

g _____ t   br _____ m   d _____ p   str _____ t

n _____ d   t _____ st   m _____ d   l _____ d

7.

wh	gh	ph

ni _____ t   _____ ony   _____ ale   _____ oto

_____ rase   _____ y   hi _____   _____ ip

8.

dd	ll	tt

le _____ uce   mi _____ le   wi _____ ow   ba _____ le

pu _____ le   bu _____ er   co _____ ar   hi _____ en

9.

pl	fl	bl

_____ ag   _____ ug   _____ end   _____ oor

_____ ease   _____ imsy   _____ ead   _____ ast

Workbook for Language Skills copyright © Susan Howell Brubaker 2009

10.

scr	str	shr

_____ ing	_____ atch	_____ ong	_____ ill
_____ ipt	_____ ain	_____ ape	_____ iek

11.

oi	ai	ui

n _____ se	g _____ lty	st _____ rs	ch _____ ce
tr _____ n	d _____ sy	q _____ ck	sq _____ rrel

12.

ice	ite	ide

dec _____ d	su _____	ev _____ nce	wa _____ r
vo _____ s	sp _____ r	l _____ nse	v _____ o

13.

tion	ness	ment

docu _____	wit _____	ce _____	vaca _____
busi _____	ele _____	ques _____	wit _____

14.

ffe	enn	cce

t _____ is	su _____ ss	di _____ rent	o _____ red
a _____ pt	co _____ e	k _____ el	so _____ r

160

TARGET AREA 3: Spelling   Words from Choices

DIRECTIONS: A list of letters is shown in each box. Put one letter from the list in each blank to form a word. Letters can be used more than once or not at all.

EXAMPLE: **r b l p c j**

_j_ a _r_   _b_ il _l_

_c_ o _p_   _p_ i _c_ k

1. **n g z b q c a h**

a ___ e   ___ ot   ___ oo

___ uit   ___ arm   ___ u ___

___ ebr ___   ___ reen   ___ rin ___

2. **q g y p b h l k**

mi ___ ___   ___ andy   ___ rave

___ a ___ er   jo ___ ing   ___ ard

___ uic ___   ___ isten   ___ a ___

3. **n f k s p t y g**

___ oo ___   wa ___ ___ e   ac ___

ea ___ ___   ___ ar ___   ___ o ___ e

co ___ ___   ri ___ ___   ___ ___ unk

Workbook for Language Skills copyright © Susan Howell Brubaker 2009

4. **c g r b t x f h**

___ o ___   s ___ a ___   ___ a ___

di ___ ___   ___ i ___ e   ___ ___ in

___ ea ___   s ___ a ___ e   ___ al ___

---

5. **i y w x o c g m**

e ___ pe ___ t   ta ___   ___ oan

f ___ ___   bu ___   e ___ tra

___ ron ___   ___ an ___   c ___ t ___

---

6. **d j l n p w s v**

___ am ___   ___ o ___   ___ ay

___ ho ___   ki ___ ___   ___ a ___ t

___ oa ___   ___ i ___ e   ___ ai ___

---

7. **a e i o u y**

tr ___ ff ___ c   m ___ n ___ ___   s ___ ns ___ bl ___

d ___ sc ___ v ___ r   h ___ rr ___   cr ___ st ___ l

___ r ___ ng ___   p ___ ___ dl ___   p ___ t ___ t

8. **c m n r s v w x**

au ___ tio ___   e ___ ade   ___ ho ___ el

fou ___ th   ___ ilita ___ y   ba ___ gai ___

___ a ___ dy   fi ___ e ___ ood   e ___ ___ ited

9. **b d j k l p t y**

ca ___ ___ ure   ___ eanu ___   hea ___ ___ h

fanc ___   ___ ung ___ e   s ___ en ___ er

___ iqui ___   ___ isso ___ ve   varie ___ ___

10. **r g h v f e x n**

___ ___ avity   t ___ ___ oat   u ___ i ___ o ___ m

ind ___ ___   le ___ e ___ d   mo ___ i ___ s

___ le ___ ible   ___ o ___ mal   ___ u ___ ious

11. **q i c a t s b z**

___ oun ___ e   gr ___ ___ n   ke ___ ___ hup

we ___ ___ thy   pri ___ e   mu ___ ___ le

be ___ ___ h   re ___ ul ___   bre ___ ___ hing

TARGET AREA 3: Spelling   Words from Clues

DIRECTIONS: In each exercise a word is described. Read the description. Put one letter in the blank to form the word.

EXAMPLE: stop doing something	qui __*t*__	
a type of test	qui __*z*__	

1. plead for something   b ___ g

   a small insect   b ___ g

   opposite of small   b ___ g

   carry groceries in it   b ___ g

2. a dog is a good one   p ___ t

   a name   P ___ t

   center of a cherry   p ___ t

   something to cook in   p ___ t

3. a very fine rain   m ___ st

   part of a sailboat   m ___ st

   opposite of least   m ___ st

   have to do something   m ___ st

4. a man's nickname   D ___ c k

    a water bird   d ___ c k

    a pack of cards   d ___ c k

    a place for boats   d ___ c k

---

5. a sharp object   p ___ n

    a writing utensil   p ___ n

    a play on words   p ___ n

    a cooking utensil   p ___ n

---

6. it lays eggs   ___ e n

    a man's name   ___ e n

    males   ___ e n

    more than nine   ___ e n

---

7. be in a hurry   ___ u s h

    type of shrubbery   ___ u s h

    be quiet   ___ u s h

    opposite of pull   ___ u s h

8. man's name   ___ ay

    like straw   ___ ay

    fifth month   ___ ay

    give money   ___ ay

---

9. kind of pickle   ___ ill

    medicine   ___ ill

    sloping land   ___ ill

    record of a sale   ___ ill

---

10. very chilly   ___ old

    already said   ___ old

    valuable metal   ___ old

    got money for   ___ old

---

11. take it easy   ___ est

    home for a bird   ___ est

    sleeveless clothing   ___ est

    better than the rest   ___ est

TARGET AREA 3: Spelling   Missing Consonants

DIRECTIONS: In each exercise a word is described. Read the description. Put one letter in each blank to form the word.

| EXAMPLE: division of a house | _r_ oo _m_ |
| what we eat | _f_ oo _d_ |

1. a plant starts from it   ___ ee ___

   take a quick look   ___ ee ___

   the back of your foot   ___ ee ___

   meat from a cow   ___ ee ___

---

2. scalp covering   ___ ai ___

   the primary one   ___ ai ___

   the opposite of **succeed**   ___ ai ___

   another word for **spoke**   ___ ai ___

---

3. 60 minutes   ___ ou ___

   very noisy   ___ ou ___

   a person, place, or thing   ___ ou ___

   food eaten from a bowl with a spoon   ___ ou ___

4. the shape of bread   ___ o a ___

     similar to a frog   ___ o a ___

     to leave in a liquid   ___ o a ___

     the top of beer or type of rubber   ___ o a ___

---

5. two people who sing together   ___ u e ___

     abbreviation for a weekday   ___ u e ___

     a source of energy like gas   ___ u e ___

     took to court   ___ u e ___

---

6. the opposite of strong   ___ e a ___

     fruit from a tree   ___ e a ___

     meat from a calf   ___ e a ___

     not able to hear   ___ e a ___

---

7. did not tell the truth   ___ i e ___

     opinion; point of _____   ___ i e ___

     guide for losing weight   ___ i e ___

     walkway going out into water   ___ i e ___

8. absolutely positive   ___ u ___ e

    the sixth month   ___ u ___ e

    a six-sided square   ___ u ___ e

    without clothing   ___ u ___ e

---

9. a contest for speed   ___ a ___ e

    opposite of **wild**   ___ a ___ e

    a ridge of water   ___ a ___ e

    a sheet from a book   ___ a ___ e

---

10. story with a punch line   ___ o ___ e

    way to elect someone   ___ o ___ e

    small burrowing animal   ___ o ___ e

    skeleton material   ___ o ___ e

---

11. side dish instead of potatoes   ___ i ___ e

    what a clock tells you   ___ i ___ e

    spouse of a husband   ___ i ___ e

    a number   ___ i ___ e

TARGET AREA 3: Spelling   Letter Addition

DIRECTIONS: Put one letter in the blank to form a word. Letters can be used more than once.

EXAMPLE: ba ___*c*___ k

A B C D E F G H I J K L M N O P Q R S T U V W X Y Z

1. gl ___ ss

2. b ___ rry

3. ___ allon

4. lea ___ e

5. poo ___

6. ___ ind

7. a ___ chor

8. se ___ en

9. ho ___ se

10. ju ___ ge

11. ___ asy

12. hab ___ t

13. puzz ___ e

14. pla ___ tic

15. bro ___ n

16. ___ nob

17. org ___ n

18. ra ___ io

19. ___ atch

20. th ___ rn

21. pyr ___ mid

22. i ___ age

23. lig ___ t

24. s ___ ared

25. rod ___ o

26. ___ erson

27. st ___ ong

28. ban ___ na

29. af ___ er

30. ca ___ p

31. d ___ ain

32. whal ___

33. blo ___ d

34. grou ___ d

35. ___ ute

36. c ___ oset

37. ali ___ e

38. ob ___ ect

39. wo ___ ld

40. con ___ ert

41. p ___ ano

42. li ___ uid

43. ta ___ k

44. sausa ___ e

TARGET AREA 3: Spelling   Specific Letter Addition

DIRECTIONS: Put one letter in each blank to form a word. Letters can be used more than once.

EXAMPLE: ch __*i*__ ck __*e*__ n

A B C D E F G H I J K L M N O P Q R S T U V W X Y Z

1. di ___ ___ icult

2. e ___ rth ___ uake

3. m ___ g ___ cian

4. ___ illio ___ aire

5. ele ___ ___ ant

6. ca ___ dida ___ e

7. in ___ ustr ___

8. scre ___ d ___ iver

9. jea ___ ou ___

10. b ___ f ___ alo

11. c ___ l ___ ry

12. apa ___ tm ___ nt

13. te ___ ep ___ one

14. ___ cc ___ pt

15. ___ umpk ___ n

16. f ___ ng ___ r

17. a ___ bula ___ ce

18. th ___ ___ sand

19. de ___ isi ___ n

20. ___ eginnin ___

21. ___ vai ___ able

22. ra ___ tles ___ ake

23. s ___ rap ___ ook

24. app ___ intm ___ nt

25. b ___ sketb ___ ll

26. ___ rapefru ___ t

27. can ___ ellatio ___

28. an ___ m ___ l

29. ___ ushio ___

30. um ___ rel ___ a

31. i ___ ___ ustrate

32. ve ___ tica ___

33. suc ___ es ___ ful

34. a ___ ___ ow

35. a ___ pha ___ et

36. ha ___ pines ___

37. p ___ otog ___ aph

38. bin ___ cu ___ ars

39. tele ___ ___ ope

40. ___ rigin ___ l

41. m ___ unta ___ n

42. ___ ecaus ___

43. ___ ympa ___ hy

44. kno ___ le ___ ge

TARGET AREA 3: Spelling   Two-Letter Additions

DIRECTIONS: Put one letter in each blank to form a word. Letters can be used more than once.

EXAMPLE: ___*h*___ or ___*n*___

A B C D E F G H I J K L M N O P Q R S T U V W X Y Z

1. ___ e a ___

2. ___ i ___ e

3. ___ o o ___

4. h ___ s ___

5. ___ o a ___

6. ___ a ___ e

7. ___ ___ s t

8. c o ___ ___

9. ___ ___ x

10. ___ ___ s h

11. ___ i r ___

12. s ___ ___ k

13. ___ e e ___

14. g r ___ ___

15. ___ ___ n g

16. ___ a i ___

17. ___ e ___ r

18. b l ___ ___

19. t h ___ ___

20. ___ i o ___

21. ___ ___ ts

22. f ___ ___ m

23. ___ ___ rt

24. w ___ ___ m

25. ___ ___ ss

26. ___ i ___ g

27. ___ ou ___

28. fl ___ ___ e

29. bo ___ ___

30. ___ i ___ t

31. ___ ___ est

32. ___ a ___ ch

33. ___ ___ ll

34. ch ___ ___

35. ___ ___ old

36. ___ os ___

37. t ___ ___ e

38. st ___ ___

39. we ___ ___

40. ___ ___ ose

41. j ___ ___ t

42. ___ u ___ e

43. s ___ o ___ e

44. wr ___ ___

TARGET AREA 3: Spelling

Word Endings

DIRECTIONS: Put one or more letters in the blank to form a word.

EXAMPLE: spe **nd,** **special**

1. rel _____

2. cor _____

3. mis _____

4. pol _____

5. rep _____

6. gal _____

7. ele _____

8. san _____

9. pre _____

10. sub _____

11. col _____

12. pas _____

13. sta _____

14. ble _____

15. shr _____

16. cou _____

17. blo _____

18. chu _____

19. des _____

20. swi _____

21. scr _____

22. all _____

23. ger _____

24. liv _____

25. ini _____

26. ove _____

27. ban _____

28. qui _____

29. rai _____

30. fro _____

31. squ _____

32. chi _____

33. joc _____

34. lan _____

35. kee _____

36. exa _____

37. tra _____

38. han _____

39. non _____

40. tac _____

41. exc _____

42. pro _____

43. gre _____

44. loc _____

TARGET AREA 3: Spelling

DIRECTIONS: *Put one or more letters in the blank to form a word.*

EXAMPLE: _____ *fi* rst   or   _____ *wo* rst

1. _____ ble

2. _____ sts

3. _____ ard

4. _____ bby

5. _____ vel

6. _____ ing

7. _____ ass

8. _____ ice

9. _____ der

10. _____ ous

11. _____ ive

12. _____ eek

13. _____ nce

14. _____ les

15. _____ tle

16. _____ ake

17. _____ rch

18. _____ esh

19. _____ iff

20. _____ own

21. _____ all

22. _____ ddy

23. _____ rip

24. _____ jor

25. _____ use

26. _____ int

27. _____ ces

28. _____ ple

29. _____ ose

30. _____ ick

31. _____ uff

32. _____ age

33. _____ yer

34. _____ eed

35. _____ ave

36. _____ ker

37. _____ ies

38. _____ ash

39. _____ ver

40. _____ ult

41. _____ yly

42. _____ ame

43. _____ wer

44. _____ rth

TARGET AREA 3: Spelling   Homonyms

DIRECTIONS: Each sentence contains a blank with a word in parentheses after it.
Write a word in the blank that sounds like the word in parentheses
but is spelled differently.

EXAMPLE: He _____***weighs***_____ (ways) 200 pounds.

---

1. The black _____ (bare) was dangerous.

2. That man has a large _____ (knows).

3. I can't decide what to _____ (ware).

4. Speak up! I can't _____ (here) very well.

5. The baby has really _____ (groan).

6. A female deer is called a _____ (dough).

7. That cabinet won't _____ (cell).

8. My car needs to be _____ (toad).

9. She _____ (war) a brown dress.

10. A yellow _____ (rows)   was in the vase.

11. The wound should _____ (he'll)   soon.

12. This is the _____ (mane)   road to Troy.

13. I'll have a _____ (pair)   for dessert.

14. I _____ (guest)   that they would get lost.

15. _____ (There)   dog's name is Rags.

16. Are you over the _____ (flew)?

17. The book was _____ (dew)   at the library.

18. I think I deserve a _____ (rays)   in pay.

19. He went _____ (threw)   the revolving door.

20. The box of _____ (serial)   fell on the floor.

21. It's not polite to _____ (stair)   at someone.

22. The vegetables _____ (knead) more salt.

23. I had to _____ (weight) a long time in line.

24. The mail was _____ (cent) to the wrong address.

25. Some cats have long _____ (fir).

26. I will _____ (meat) you by the main entrance.

27. Of _____ (coarse), I'll go with you.

28. A gun will _____ (chute) bullets.

29. I'd like some _____ (piece) and quiet.

30. The car needs new _____ (breaks).

31. I _____ (one) first

_____ (pries).

32. The wind _____ (blue)

my _____ (hare).

TARGET AREA 3: Spelling   Guided Words

DIRECTIONS: Write a word on the line that fits the description.

EXAMPLE: Write a word with 2 syllables in it.

broken

---

1. Write a word made of 2 smaller words put together.

_____

2. Write a word with **TH** in it. _____

3. Write a word with two **O**'s in it. _____

4. Write a word that ends in **E**. _____

5. Write a word that begins with **D** and ends with **K**.

_____

6. Write a word that begins with **S** and ends with **E**.

_____

7. Write a word that begins and ends with the same letter.

_____

8. Write a word that begins with **STR**. _____

9. Write a word with 6 letters in it. _____

10. Write a word that has the same letter in it three times.

   _____

11. Write a word that is always capitalized. _____

12. Write a contraction (example: don't). _____

13. Write a word that has a **Z** in it. _____

14. Write two words that are pronounced alike but spelled

   differently. _____   _____

15. Write a word with two or more **S**'s in it. _____

16. Write the longest word you can think of.

   _____

17. Write 2 two-letter words.

   _____   _____

18. Write a word that has an **F, G,** or **H** in it.

   _____

Workbook for Language Skills copyright © Susan Howell Brubaker 2009

19. Write a word that begins with **EX**. _____

20. Write a word with **QU** in it. _____

21. Write a word that rhymes with **dough**. _____

22. Write a word with at least eight letters in it.

_____

23. Write a word that has two **M**'s in it. _____

24. Write a word that has a **PL** in it. _____

25. Write a word that has a double **B** in it.

_____

26. Write a word that does not have an **S** at the end when it is plural.

_____

27. Write a word that ends in **CH**. _____

28. Write a word that has an **F** in it but does not start with **F**.

_____

TARGET AREA 4:
Completions—Open

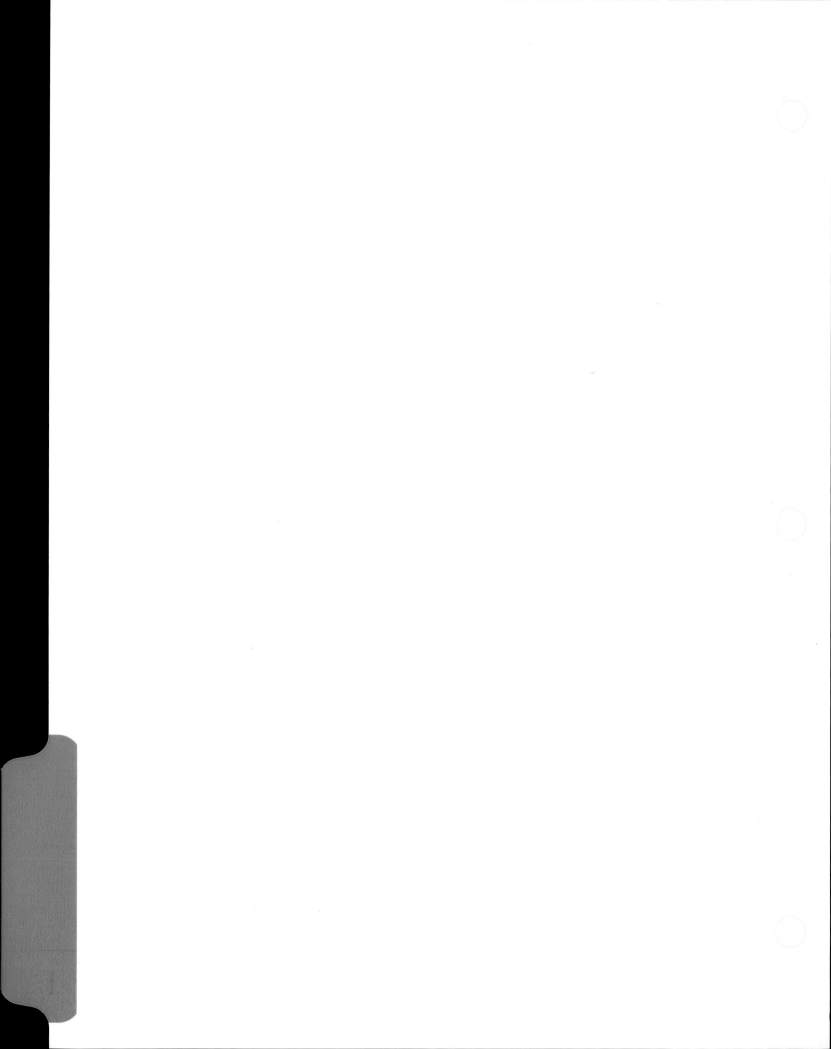

TARGET AREA 4: Completions — Open   General—One Word

DIRECTIONS: *Think of a word that makes sense in the sentence and write it on the line.*

EXAMPLE: The plant needs light and ___*water*___ .

---

1. It's disturbing to see _____ thrown along the highways.

---

2. I talked to the _____ and made an appointment to see the dentist on Friday.

---

3. The Democratic Party had a fund-raising _____ last night.

---

4. You must have your _____ before you can get a refund on the item.

---

5. The punch for the party would not be complete without _____ .

---

6. He left his dirty shirts at the _____ .

7. They rushed her to the _____ because she was

   having chest pains.

   _____

8. _____ need special equipment to do their

   job properly.

   _____

9. _____ is good exercise.

   _____

10. The score was _____ so the game went

    into overtime.

    _____

11. We have enough grape jelly, but we need more _____ .

    _____

12. It would be easier to cut off the branches if I had a

    better _____ .

    _____

13. The Saturday night _____ League will not meet

    this week.

    _____

14. Throw out the _____ ; it looks moldy.

    _____

15. The nurse checked her pulse and her _____

    pressure reading.

16. She would look better if she got a _____ .

17. I have enough yarn to _____ a sweater.

18. Their political views are more _____ than mine.

19. Sometimes I order a _____ salad for lunch.

20. The dog needed a rabies _____ .

21. He rested his feet on the _____ .

22. His _____ was dripping with perspiration.

23. The Post Office requires a _____ code on letters
    to help get them delivered.

24. She is a junior _____ in the law firm.

25. Although the criminal was sentenced to five years, he was a model
    prisoner and got _____ in two years.

26. The audience _____ loudly at the end of

the performance.

27. The club raised over $6,000 for _____ research.

28. The old mansion had a beautiful winding _____

to the second floor.

29. The freezer has an automatic _____ so you don't

have to clean out the ice yourself.

30. He aimed, but he didn't squeeze the _____ .

31. I looked in every _____ of my desk, but I can't

find a stapler.

32. You can't park in front of a fire _____ .

33. The _____ to the lodge were easy to follow.

34. They took a _____ instead of driving to Chicago.

TARGET AREA 4: Completions — Open   Phrases

DIRECTIONS: Add one or more words to the words listed to form a familiar phrase.

EXAMPLE: run   *of the mill,   run away*

1. blue _____

2. fried _____

3. snow _____

4. roll _____

5. Eiffel _____

6. Lake _____

7. Coney _____

8. eye _____

9. North _____

10. foot _____

192

11. New _____

12. chocolate _____

13. green _____

14. double _____

15. ice _____

16. blood _____

17. credit _____

18. down _____

19. red _____

20. long _____

21. United _____

22. over _____

23. sun _____

24. heart _____

25. old _____

26. good _____

27. barbecue _____

28. light _____

29. high _____

30. last _____

31. air _____

32. hand _____

33. water _____

34. public _____

35. triple _____

36. middle _____

TARGET AREA 4: Completions — Open   General—Two Words

DIRECTIONS: Each sentence is incomplete. Think of words that would make sense in the sentence, and write them on the lines.

EXAMPLE: He ran from one end of the _____*field*_____

to the _____*other*_____ .

1. Our weekly _____ game was postponed

   until _____ .

_____

2. The _____ was introduced, and the audience

   began to _____ .

_____

3. The _____ took two orders for hot

   fudge _____ .

_____

4. He was _____ when he heard

   the _____ .

_____

5. The Johnsons are moving to _____ because of its

   good _____ .

6. I shut and _____ the door before I

_____ the house.

7. She is the _____ woman I have

ever _____ .

8. I'm so _____ that I think I could

_____ for a week.

9. I defrosted _____ and I will heat up some

_____ for dinner.

10. _____ is a great _____ .

11. The new national _____ champion was honored

at a private _____ .

12. I can't catch the _____ because when I get close,

it runs under the _____ .

13. The _____ tastes like _____ .

14. I made a dozen _____ muffins and bought a

    dozen _____ doughnuts for the brunch.

---

15. The hot _____ burned

    my _____ .

---

16. Jason and his _____ live in a

    _____ in Vermont.

---

17. The average _____ spends eight hours a

    day _____ .

---

18. The _____ of a rabbit is

    very _____ .

---

19. It is illegal to _____ when you

    are _____ .

---

20. After the lawn has been _____ , then you can

    _____ it.

21. The _____ tripped and dropped a

_____ on me.

22. The _____ were born _____

weeks early.

23. Anna _____ loudly when she heard

the _____ .

24. You bring the _____ and I'll make a

_____ for the party.

25. Jill joined a _____ so she could lose _____ .

26. _____ piled up on the _____

while they were gone.

27. The _____ tasted very bland so I added

some _____ .

28. Every morning I take my _____ before I have

some _____ .

TARGET AREA 4: Completions — Open   General—Multiple Words

DIRECTIONS: Write several words to complete each sentence.

EXAMPLE: The bill for this month's installment was _____

_____ *due on the fifteenth.* _____

---

1. The president spoke with _____

_____

2. Finally I found _____

_____

3. The picnic lasted _____

_____

4. Instead of being where they usually are, the keys were _____

_____

5. About the only thing a dollar can buy today is _____

_____

6. The first person who arrives should _____

_____

7. The music tonight will be provided by _____

   _____

8. The shoes needed repair because _____

   _____

9. The judge demanded that _____

   _____

10. I left the laundry _____

    _____

11. The people were in line _____

    _____

12. Stock prices plunged _____

    _____

13. They were whispering _____

    _____

14. The price of food is _____

    _____

15. With her eyes closed, she _____

_____

16. We listened for the _____

_____

17. The union strike lasted _____

_____

18. By the age of 16, most boys _____

_____

19. Where can you get _____

_____

20. The electrician finished wiring the _____

_____

21. The hotel guests were concerned when _____

_____

22. Discount tickets are available for _____

_____

23. After he got a loan, he _____

_____

24. The judge explained that _____

_____

25. Even though it was raining, the _____

_____

26. The Board of Directors meets monthly to _____

_____

27. After I scraped off the paint _____

_____

28. On Sunday afternoon they went to _____

_____

29. The illegal drugs were found in _____

_____

30. Many people felt the election was _____

_____

31. I found the stray _____

_____

32. The UPS driver brought _____

_____

33. After the half-time show, _____

_____

34. The broken shells hurt _____

_____

35. At the cider mill you could _____

_____

36. Every day I make sure I _____

_____

37. Local businesses were asked to _____

_____

38. Each year consumers spend millions on _____

_____

TARGET AREA 4: Completions — Open   Opinions

DIRECTIONS: Write several words to complete each sentence.

> EXAMPLE: One of these days, *I'll take a vacation.*

1. When I feel angry, I _____

_____

2. The nice thing about a rainy day is _____

_____

3. Without much effort I could _____

_____

4. Getting older isn't so bad because _____

_____

5. I wish I had the time to _____

_____

6. The best thing I ever did for myself was _____

_____

7. My biggest frustration is _____

_____

8. I smile when I think about _____

_____

9. We live in a historic time because _____

_____

10. I envy people who _____

_____

11. I think of my father when _____

_____

12. The first thing in the morning I am _____

_____

13. I hope to be remembered for my _____

_____

14. The nicest present I could get would be _____

_____

15. I get upset when _____

_____

16. The best thing about me is _____

_____

17. I like to _____

_____

18. I strongly believe that _____

_____

19. I would like to win a _____

_____

20. I hope someday I will find _____

_____

21. As a child, I really liked to _____

_____

22. I like to be alone when _____

_____

23. I would like to forget _____

_____

24. Someone who is very important to me is _____

_____

25. If I were invisible, _____

_____

26. This is a good day for me to _____

_____

27. I'm so glad someone invented _____

_____

28. I don't like to think about _____

_____

29. I'm proud of myself when _____

_____

30. It's hard for me to admit that _____

_____

31. I don't know what I would do without _____

_____

32. I know it's important to _____

_____

33. I am impressed with _____

_____

34. I get a lot of pleasure from _____

_____

35. I enjoy having _____

_____

36. My comfort food is _____

_____

37. If I didn't have TV, I would _____

_____

38. The best pet I knew was _____

_____

TARGET AREA 4: Completions — Open   Factual Statements

DIRECTIONS: Write several words to complete each sentence.

EXAMPLE: People use credit cards when ___*they don't*___

___*have any cash with them.*___

1. Streets have sewers so that _____

_____

2. Charitable organizations ask for donations because _____

_____

3. Reducing the amount of salt you eat will _____

_____

4. On ebay.com you can _____

_____

5. An advantage of a cell phone or iphone is _____

_____

6. Someone may be in a wheelchair because _____

_____

7. A copyright protects _____

_____

8. You might develop a headache after you _____

_____

9. Chicken should be thoroughly cooked so _____

_____

10. A high credit score can help you _____

_____

11. The Salvation Army helps _____

_____

12. Someone might hire a detective to _____

_____

13. Some car accidents are caused by _____

_____

14. Flowers are nice to send when _____

_____

15. Parents should not allow their children to _____

_____

16. Home prices are lower when _____

_____

17. You might get a sore throat from _____

_____

18. Illegible handwriting can be a problem when _____

_____

19. In a thunderstorm, do not _____

_____

20. Wash your hands before _____

_____

21. Underage drinking can result in _____

_____

22. You can be arrested for _____

_____

23. You should go to an emergency center if _____

_____

24. Common allergies people have are _____

_____

25. People put paintings on their walls because _____

_____

26. Digital cameras allow you to _____

_____

27. An advantage of renting movies is _____

_____

28. Hardwood floors are popular because _____

_____

29. Some people want fences around their property to _____

_____

30. College scholarships are offered for _____

_____

31. The stock market fluctuates _____

_____

32. The price of a car is high because _____

_____

33. Lobster is hard to eat because _____

_____

34. People make wills so that _____

_____

35. You would want to stop payment on a check if _____

_____

36. Some superstitions are _____

_____

37. Sales help retail stores by _____

_____

38. July 4th celebrates the _____

_____

TARGET AREA 5:
Formulation

TARGET AREA 5: Formulation   Word Substitution

DIRECTIONS: Below each sentence in a group are three words in parentheses. Substitute the first word in parentheses for a word in the sentence, and rewrite the sentence. Then substitute the second word in parentheses for another word in your second sentence, and rewrite that. Continue in the same way for the third word in parentheses.

EXAMPLE: The man had new shoes.

(woman)   *The woman had new shoes.*

(earrings)   *The woman had new earrings.*

(wore)   *The woman wore new earrings.*

---

1. John Smith is running for governor.

   (mayor)   _____

   (Steven)   _____

   (voting)   _____

---

2. The brown couch is by the wall.

   (window)   _____

   (oak cabinet)   _____

   (across from)   _____

3. The dog chewed the bone.

(shoe) _____

(dropped) _____

(man) _____

4. Would you like a piece of pie?

(apple) _____

(tuna sandwich) _____

(did you have) _____

5. The woman has a basket of yellow roses.

(He) _____

(bouquet) _____

(tulips) _____

6. A mug of beer is on the table.

(counter) _____

(cup of coffee) _____

(jar) _____

7. The flight to Chicago was full.

   (delayed) _____

   (New York) _____

   (bus) _____

8. Niagara Falls is a nice place for a honeymoon.

   (vacation) _____

   (Disneyland) _____

   (family) _____

9. The baby's rattle was under the sofa.

   (TV) _____

   (bottle) _____

   (next to) _____

10. The symphony gave a concert on Thursday.

    (singer) _____

    (Saturday) _____

    (party) _____

11. The horse trotted into the corral.

    (walked back) _____

    (barn) _____

    (cow) _____

12. A pleasant clerk showed me a coat.

    (sold) _____

    (area rug) _____

    (busy) _____

13. I ordered a salad for lunch.

    (hamburger) _____

    (cooked) _____

    (my friend) _____

14. It was a cold day for a football game.

    (good) _____

    (tennis match) _____

    (Thursday) _____

15. The chickadee chirped in the elm tree.

    (perched) _____

    (owl hooted) _____

    (maple) _____

16. Would you like a pizza after the concert?

    (before) _____

    (drink) _____

    (movie) _____

17. The gray wool carpet was new.

    (suit) _____

    (linen) _____

    (red) _____

18. Cars have radios and trees have branches.

    (engines) _____

    (leaves) _____

    (trains) _____

TARGET AREA 5: Formulation   Sentence Combination

DIRECTIONS: Each group has two short sentences. Combine the two sentences into one, and write the new sentence. Make the new sentence as short as you can but include the facts.

EXAMPLE: A dog walked by. It was a black dog.

A black dog walked by.

---

1. It was a cloudy afternoon. It was cool. It was breezy.

_____

_____

2. That man is my boss. He is wearing a brown suit.

_____

_____

3. The movie is about two sisters. They are twins.

_____

_____

4. Lettuce is on sale this week. Onions and bananas are also on sale.

_____

_____

5. I would like to see a pair of slippers. I need size 8.

_____

_____

6. The batter hit the ball. It was a home run.

_____

_____

7. The baby is hungry. The baby is crying.

_____

_____

8. There was a package on the front steps. FedEx delivered it.

_____

_____

9. Your coat has a stain on it. It needs to be cleaned.

_____

_____

10. It is windy outside. Papers and leaves are blowing in the street.

_____

_____

11. Many adults continue their education. Some take night classes.

_____

_____

12. He tripped. A dog toy was the cause. He broke his ankle.

_____

_____

13. Some people listen to music. Music can be relaxing.

_____

_____

14. A sale starts on Tuesday. The sale is on winter coats. The sale is today.

_____

_____

15. I shop at Oakwood Mall. The mall is close to my home.

_____

_____

16. There was a car accident. It was on the corner. It involved three cars.

_____

_____

17. Today is Bob Martin's birthday. He is 50 years old.

_____

_____

18. This house has three bedrooms. It has two bathrooms. It is a ranch.

_____

_____

19. The ice cream is melted. The freezer is not working properly.

_____

_____

20. Last month Les went hunting. He shot two pheasants. He missed four.

_____

_____

21. Fresh flowers can be bought at the florist. You can buy plants there too.

_____

_____

22. The boy climbed a tree. He fell. He broke his leg in two places.

_____

_____

23. Chevrolet for sale: It is a Tahoe. It is in excellent condition. It is blue.

_____

_____

24. A black dog growled at another dog. The other dog was a brown-and-white terrier. The black dog was small. The other dog was larger.

_____

_____

25. He ordered a chocolate sundae. He wanted whipped cream on it. He did not want nuts.

_____

_____

26. I poured myself a cup of tea. I poured a cup for Barb. It was green tea.

_____

_____

27. There is a bowl of fruit. There is a banana in the bowl. The bowl is on the table. Apples and pears are in the bowl.

_____

_____

TARGET AREA 5: Formulation   Abbreviation Expansion

DIRECTIONS: Each sentence contains some abbreviations. Rewrite the sentence and spell out all the abbreviations.

EXAMPLE: The Dr.'s bill was $45.00.

The doctor's bill was forty-five dollars.

---

1. Col. Smith works in the 1st bldg. on the blvd.

   _____

   _____

2. The address is 430 Oak Ave., St. Louis, MO.

   _____

   _____

3. Your next appt. is on Tues., Nov. 3, @ 2:30.

   _____

   _____

4. Maple Rd. is 2 mi. on your rt.

   _____

   _____

226

5. The pkg. weighed 47 lbs. 3½ oz.

_____

_____

6. Mr. Wm. Day Jr. is an atty.

_____

_____

7. Eggs cost $2.89/doz and milk costs $2.39 a ½ gal.

_____

_____

8. 3 ft. = 1 yd.

_____

_____

9. He received a BS from MSU.

_____

_____

10. The mgr. hired an ass't. on Mon.

_____

_____

11. The temp. is 72°F in NYC.

_____

_____

12. It is 4 mo. til X-mas.

_____

_____

13. L.A. is the 2nd largest city in the USA.

_____

_____

14. The apt. has 1,500 sq. ft., DR, and a FP.

_____

_____

15. Dr. Kelly of the FBI called Gen. Hicks of the CIA.

_____

_____

16. The recipe called for 2 c. + 3 t. sugar.

_____

_____

228

17. My SUV gets about 30 mpg when traveling at 55 mph.

_____

_____

18. Sales tax in FL. is 6%.

_____

_____

19. CT. is NE of TX.

_____

_____

20. Prof. Snyder is hd. of the gov't. dept.

_____

_____

21. The order was a BLT on rye, a Dr. Pepper, and Fr. fries.

_____

_____

22. The EC is near the RR crossing on Hwy. 62.

_____

_____

TARGET AREA 5: Formulation　　　　　　　　Sentence Construction

DIRECTIONS: Write one sentence using all the words in each group. You can use the words in any order.

EXAMPLE: sitting, chair, brown

I am sitting on a brown chair.

---

1. turn, light, bathroom _____

_____

2. toss, lettuce, blue cheese _____

_____

3. take, blanket, cleaners _____

_____

4. arrange, roses, vase _____

_____

5. TV, special, tonight _____

_____

6. I, chair, sale _____

_____

7. pick, bushel, pears _____

_____

8. wash, trim, hair _____

_____

9. walk, mile, later _____

_____

10. sand, hot, beach _____

_____

11. cookies, baking, oven _____

_____

12. uncle, born, Iowa _____

_____

13. there, spider, wall _____

_____

14. sleep, holiday, tomorrow _____

_____

15. want, stock, price _____

_____

16. two, schedule, train _____

_____

17. the, cracked, edge _____

_____

18. do, know, going _____

_____

19. put, lid, jam _____

_____

20. parrot, unusual, colorful _____

_____

21. call, fire, kitchen _____

_____

22. let's, chicken, out _____

_____

232

23. surgery, donor, kidney _____

_____

24. basketball, taller, score _____

_____

25. star, sing, country _____

_____

26. listen, attend, lecture _____

_____

27. work, hard, succeed _____

_____

28. bottle, floating, ocean _____

_____

29. pleasant, tour, city _____

_____

30. erase, mistakes, puzzle _____

_____

TARGET AREA 5: Formulation   Rephrase Idioms

DIRECTIONS: Replace the underlined phrase in each sentence with other words that mean about the same thing. Rewrite the new sentence. You may also need to change the wording of the sentence when you rewrite it.

EXAMPLE: She <u>dropped out of</u> college to get hitched.

She left college so she could marry.

1. He was **tied up** all day in meetings.

_____

_____

2. It is the most **laid-back mellow** pup I have seen.

_____

_____

3. Learning to use my new camera was a **piece of cake**.

_____

_____

4. You get more **bang for your buck** by buying in bulk.

_____

_____

5. I was going to ride the coaster but I **chickened out**.

_____

_____

6. Minor repairs are **right up my alley**.

_____

_____

7. They were **packed like sardines** in the elevator.

_____

_____

8. I had **a lump in my throat** during the eulogy.

_____

_____

9. They are like **two peas in a pod**.

_____

_____

10. If you weren't such a **party animal**, you wouldn't be so **hung over**.

_____

_____

11. We drove for two hours before making a **pit stop**.

_____

_____

12. That commercial **drives me up a wall**.

_____

_____

13. He **lost his shirt** gambling in Las Vegas.

_____

_____

14. **Stick with it**—you've **got the smarts** to do the job.

_____

_____

15. The comedian had **butterflies in his stomach** before his performance.

_____

_____

16. He is **hot under the collar** because I **beat him to** the interview.

_____

17. You are **off the hook**—I found a babysitter.

_____

_____

18. **Once in a blue moon**, I buy a lottery ticket.

_____

_____

19. Your sister has **a heart of gold**.

_____

_____

20. He **lost his cool** and offended a **long-time** customer.

_____

_____

21. I was **bummed out** that I didn't get picked.

_____

_____

22. **Here's the deal**—**hit the books** for an hour and then you can watch TV.

_____

_____

TARGET AREA 5: Formulation   Response to an Encounter

DIRECTIONS: In each group somebody is saying something. Write what you would say in response to that person if he or she were speaking to you.

EXAMPLE: **Police officer:** May I see your driver's license?

Yes, just a moment while I get it.

1. **Clerk:** Is this cash or charge?

2. **Waitress:** May I take your order, please?

3. **Clerk:** We have an incredible deal on digital cameras until Tuesday.

4. **Religious person:** The end of the world is near.

5. **Someone on the street:** Haven't I seen you in the movies?

6. **Dentist:** You need two teeth pulled.

238

7. **Drive-thru window:** Welcome to McDonald's. May I take your order?

_____

8. **Doctor:** You are 40 pounds overweight.

_____

9. **Ice cream store server:** What would you like?

_____

10. **Person on phone:** You have been chosen to receive a free overnight stay at the fabulous new . . .

_____

11. **Solicitor:** Will you sign the petition for this worthy cause?

_____

12. **Plumber:** This pipe needs to be replaced or it will burst.

_____

13. **Boss:** You have been doing an excellent job.

_____

14. **Small child:** May I have five dollars?

_____

15. **Salesperson:** I'm sorry, we are out of your size.

_____

16. **Librarian:** May I help you find something?

_____

17. **Mechanic:** It looks like the engine needs a tune-up.

_____

18. **Politician:** What can I do to get your vote?

_____

19. **Strolling musician:** What would you like to hear?

_____

20. **Art teacher:** You have a natural talent for drawing.

_____

21. **Police officer:** You were doing 40 in a 25-mile zone.

_____

22. **Teacher:** Your child is failing English.

_____

23. **Neighbor:** May I borrow your lawnmower?

_____

24. **Jockey:** He's the fastest horse on the track.

_____

25. **Friend:** What do you want to do tonight?

_____

26. **Psychic:** I see money in your future.

_____

27. **Man on the street:** I'll sell you this watch for an unbelievably low price.

_____

28. **Chef:** I will prepare whatever you desire.

_____

29. **Pharmacist:** Your prescription has expired.

_____

30. **Hotel clerk:** I'm sorry; all of our rooms are taken.

_____

TARGET AREA 5: Formulation

Question Formulation

*DIRECTIONS: In each group an Answer (A) is given to some Question (Q). Think of a question that would fit the answer and write it on the **Q** line.*

EXAMPLE: **Q:** *What time is it?*

A: Six-thirty.

1. **Q:** _____

   A: Fine, thanks.

2. **Q:** _____

   A: Warm, about 70 degrees.

3. **Q:** _____

   A: A hot dog with mustard.

4. **Q:** _____

   A: I didn't do it.

5. **Q:** _____

   A: One hundred dollars.

6. **Q:** _____

   A: First Monday in September.

7. **Q:** _____

   A: Not a chance.

8. **Q:** _____

   A: San Francisco

9. **Q:** _____

   A: I'd love to.

10. **Q:** _____

   A: Every four years.

11. **Q:** _____

   A: Grande vanilla nonfat latte.

12. **Q:** _____

   A: I don't know.

13. **Q:** _____

    A: Whenever it's convenient for you.

---

14. **Q:** _____

    A: Aphasia.

---

15. **Q:** _____

    A: Not tonight, I have a headache.

---

16. **Q:** _____

    A: Medium rare, please.

---

17. **Q:** _____

    A: Our presidential suite.

---

18. **Q:** _____

    A: The Grand Canyon.

---

19. **Q:** _____

    A: A service representative will be with you shortly.

20. **Q:** _____

    A: The 6 o'clock news.

---

21. **Q:** _____

    A: Page 98.

---

22. **Q:** _____

    A: I do.

---

23. **Q:** _____

    A: February 14th.

---

24. **Q:** _____

    A: People Magazine.

---

25. **Q:** _____

    A: It's none of your business.

---

26. **Q:** _____

    A: Six pounds eight ounces and sixteen inches long.

27. **Q:** _____

    A: Thursday.

28. **Q:** _____

    A: Ice cream and cake.

29. **Q:** _____

    A: Whenever I can.

30. **Q:** _____

    A: The check is in the mail.

31. **Q:** _____

    A: It's too hot.

32. **Q:** _____

    A: I'll do it after dinner.

33. **Q:** _____

    A: It could be the battery.

TARGET AREA 5: Formulation   Solution to a Situation

DIRECTIONS: A situation that you might face is described. Write a sentence explaining what you would say or do if you were in that situation.

> EXAMPLE: The mailman delivers a letter to you that belongs next door.
>
> *I would take the letter over to my neighbor.*

1. You are served spaghetti, but you ordered a hamburger.

   _____

   _____

2. You witness a robbery.

   _____

   _____

3. You want a raise in pay.

   _____

   _____

4. You find a kitten in a box on your doorstep.

   _____

   _____

5. A drink is spilled on you at a party.

_____

_____

6. You drop and break a valuable crystal vase.

_____

_____

7. Someone delivers a pizza that you didn't order.

_____

_____

8. Someone tries to sell you real estate over the telephone.

_____

_____

9. Someone near you chokes on a piece of food.

_____

_____

10. Someone asks you for money to buy a cup of coffee.

_____

_____

11. You feel like you are going to faint.

_____

_____

12. An IRS agent wants to meet with you.

_____

_____

13. You are hungry and feel light-headed.

_____

_____

14. You drop a chicken as you are taking it out of the oven.

_____

_____

15. At 11 pm you realize you have forgotten to take your medications today.

_____

_____

16. One side of a fingernail breaks below the quick.

_____

_____

17. Dinner is ready but your four guests have not yet arrived.

_____

_____

18. You think you sprained your ankle when you tripped.

_____

_____

19. You see a 50-dollar bill on the floor in a store.

_____

_____

20. Your wife/mother asks if she looks fat in her new outfit.

_____

_____

21. You forget a close friend's birthday.

_____

_____

22. Someone you don't like invites you for Thanksgiving dinner.

_____

_____

23. You are not able to attend your favorite niece's wedding.

_____

_____

24. A good friend asks you to support a cause that you don't agree with.

_____

_____

25. You lose more money in a card game than you have with you.

_____

_____

26. It has been hours and you cannot get to sleep.

_____

_____

27. It sounds like there is a bird or small animal caught in your chimney.

_____

_____

28. You believe you have some valuable antique family pieces.

_____

_____

TARGET AREA 5: Formulation   Paraphrase Information

DIRECTIONS: Each sentence in this exercise can be written in a different and simpler way and still mean the same thing. Rewrite each sentence in your own words so it is shorter and easier to understand.

EXAMPLE: The matron refused to converse with representatives of

the media. *The lady wouldn't talk to*

the reporters.

---

1. All at once, the music ceased.

_____

_____

2. He located a soft seat and lowered himself into it.

_____

_____

3. She donned an old garment and hustled out the door.

_____

_____

4. She gathered colorful horticultural specimens for the bouquet.

_____

_____

5. The instructions were difficult to comprehend.

_____

_____

6. The head person chatted with the laborers.

_____

_____

7. An ordinance forbids throwing refuse on public thoroughfares.

_____

_____

8. It began as a minor altercation but escalated.

_____

_____

9. He proceeded briskly to avoid the chill of the evening.

_____

_____

10. Our sojourn extended four days beyond our expectation.

_____

_____

11. It was my impression that he had concluded his presentation.

_____

_____

12. He focused on her multiple and pleasing physical attributes.

_____

_____

13. A wood barricade surrounding their abode assures them privacy.

_____

_____

14. This incessant turmoil makes my head throb.

_____

_____

15. The impudent youth was rebuked.

_____

_____

16. This oversized edifice was erected in record time with shoddy materials.

_____

_____

17. The notorious celebrity alluded to his impending incarceration.

_____

_____

18. The hors d'oeuvres were tasty and plentiful.

_____

_____

19. Regarding possible employment—we are not currently taking resumés.

_____

_____

20. He was infuriated by the trivial error.

_____

_____

21. The compassionate nurse comforted the distraught patient.

_____

_____

22. The bottle struck the pavement with such force it shattered.

_____

_____

23. He seemed astonished that I could have generated such a plausible solution.

_____

_____

24. Her attire was inappropriate for the occasion.

_____

_____

25. The tournament was terminated due to inclement weather.

_____

_____

26. Even as spectators were filling the stadium, the decision on whether the quarterback would participate was pending.

_____

_____

27. This area enjoys moderate temperatures with an abundance of precipitation during the spring months.

_____

_____

TARGET AREA 6:
Word Retrieval

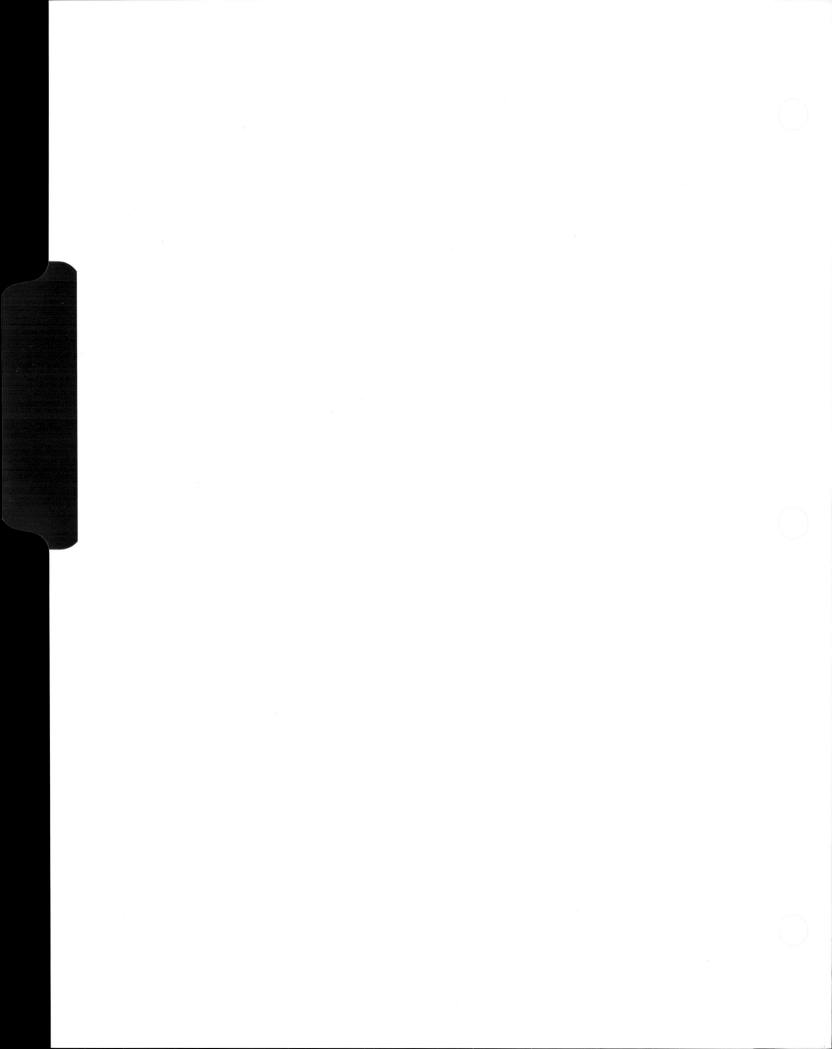

TARGET AREA 6: Word Retrieval   Matching Attributes

DIRECTIONS: The four numbered words in each item can be associated with one or more of the nine things listed below them. In front of each of the nine things, write the number of the word it refers to.

EXAMPLE: 1. candy   2. drink   3. bread   4. dessert

___*1*___ Baby Ruth   ___*4*___ cake   ___*3*___ rye

___*2*___ coke   ___*2*___ milk   ___*1*___ M & M's

1. red   2. yellow   3. blue   4. green

_____ grass   _____ lemon   _____ cardinal

_____ peas   _____ sun   _____ sky

_____ corn   _____ stop   _____ blood

1. New Orleans   2. Hollywood   3. Alaska   4. Hawaii

_____ movie star   _____ Bourbon St.   _____ Mardi Gras

_____ MGM   _____ snow   _____ luau

_____ Mt. McKinley _____ pineapple   _____ Rodeo Dr.

1. John	2. Joe	3. Jack	4. James

_____ Nicholson   _____ Montana   _____ Travolta

_____ Brown   _____ McCain   _____ Bond

_____ Hancock   _____ Sprat   _____ Biden

---

1. vegetable	2. fruit	3. meat	4. cheese

_____ artichoke   _____ muenster   _____ mango

_____ knackwurst   _____ veal   _____ parmesan

_____ sprouts   _____ yam   _____ fig

---

1. Easter	2. Christmas	3. 4th of July	4. Halloween

_____ wreath   _____ pumpkin   _____ colored egg

_____ fireworks   _____ picnic   _____ trick-or-treat

_____ bunny   _____ Santa   _____ ghost

---

1. movie	2. cartoon	3. comics	4. fairy tale

_____ Ziggy   _____ Bullwinkle   _____ Red Riding Hood

_____ Titantic   _____ Cinderella   _____ Snow White

_____ Peanuts   _____ Bugs Bunny   _____ Lion King

1. fur	2. hair	3. feathers	4. scales

_____ skunk   _____ woodpecker   _____ toddler

_____ cat   _____ wig   _____ squirrel

_____ trout   _____ peacock   _____ goldfish

---

1. movie	2. song	3. TV show	4. play

_____ Amazing Grace   _____ Good Morning America

_____ Meet the Press   _____ Blue Moon

_____ Casablanca   _____ Macbeth

_____ Sesame Street   _____ Jaws

---

1. author	2. musician	3. actor	4. politician

_____ Andrea Bocelli   _____ George Clooney

_____ Nancy Pelosi   _____ Danielle Steele

_____ Charles Dickens   _____ Kate Winslet

_____ Barack Obama   _____ Harry Connick Jr.

TARGET AREA 6: Word Retrieval   Personal Information

DIRECTIONS: Write the information asked for on the line.

EXAMPLE: Your favorite color _____ *blue* _____

1. your bank _____

2. your birthday _____

3. place where you were born _____

4. today's date _____

5. the make and year of your car _____

6. the county you live in _____

7. your mayor _____

8. your address _____

9. your phone number _____

10. your doctor's name _____

11. your Social Security number   _____

12. your parents' first names   _____

13. your middle name   _____

14. a friend's name   _____

15. your shoe size   _____

16. your height   _____

17. your eye color   _____

18. your nickname   _____

19. your dentist's name   _____

20. your insurance company name   _____

21. an organization you belong to   _____

22. a credit card you have   _____

23. a relative's name   _____

24. your next of kin _____

25. a neighbor's name _____

26. a magazine you read _____

27. your city _____

28. your zip code _____

29. your hair color _____

30. your toothpaste _____

31. a street you lived on _____

32. a pet's name _____

33. your mother's maiden name _____

34. a childhood friend _____

35. your senator _____

TARGET AREA 6: Word Retrieval

DIRECTIONS: Read each question, then write the answer on the line.

EXAMPLE: Where would you look at a menu?

at a restaurant _____

---

1. Where would you go to look at paintings?

_____

2. Where would you go to "get away from it all"?

_____

3. Where would you go to see a football game?

_____

4. Where is food served to people who are standing in line?

_____

5. Where do the president and first lady live?

_____

6. Where do you find gravestones?

_____

7. Where do you get refills of a prescription?

_____

8. Where is Washington, D.C.?

_____

9. Where do you usually buy shoes?

_____

10. Where do you board dogs?

_____

11. Where are money and valuables kept in a bank?

_____

12. Where do pro sports players go to take showers and change clothes?

_____

13. Where would you go to buy a new oven?

_____

14. Where do you find a jury?

_____

15. Where do you find a silo?

_____

16. Where is your favorite spot to sit in your home?

_____

17. Where do you keep a pair of scissors?

_____

18. Where can you buy a warm pair of gloves?

_____

19. Where do you keep ice cream?

_____

20. Where could you go to ride a roller coaster?

_____

21. Where do you put empty bottles and cans?

_____

22. Where do you keep your shampoo?

_____

TARGET AREA 6: Word Retrieval

Brand Names

DIRECTIONS: The words listed are all familiar things that we buy. Write a specific brand name next to each product.

EXAMPLE: cosmetics *Revlon, Clinique*

1. toothpaste _____

2. ice cream _____

3. shoes _____

4. coffee _____

5. beer _____

6. cheese _____

7. frozen food _____

8. soup _____

9. cereal _____

10. dog or cat food _____

11. butter or margarine _____

12. soft drink _____

13. candy bar _____

14. television set _____

15. board game _____

16. magazine _____

17. camera _____

18. aspirin _____

19. shampoo _____

20. newspaper _____

21. washer or dryer _____

22. gasoline _____

23. car _____

24. deodorant _____

25. soap _____

26. athletic shoes _____

27. toilet paper _____

28. yogurt _____

29. baked goods _____

30. luggage _____

31. pizza _____

32. mattress _____

33. tools _____

34. lightbulbs _____

35. computer _____

36. china _____

TARGET AREA 6: Word Retrieval

Local Places

DIRECTIONS: Write the name of a place in <u>your</u> neighborhood that fits each description.

EXAMPLE: a clothing store ___*The Gap*___

---

1. a restaurant _____

2. a hardware store _____

3. a church _____

4. a bakery _____

5. a fast-food place _____

6. a department store _____

7. an intersection _____

8. a popular hangout _____

9. a movie theater _____

10. a hotel _____

11. a bank _____

12. a salon or spa _____

13. a specialty shop _____

14. a furniture store _____

15. an ice cream store _____

16. a sporting goods store _____

17. a bookstore _____

18. a school _____

19. a hospital _____

20. a park _____

21. an organization _____

22. a drugstore _____

23. a jewelry store _____

24. a gas station _____

25. a grocery store _____

26. a pet store _____

27. a river _____

28. a main highway _____

29. a delicatessen _____

30. a discount store _____

31. a movie theater _____

32. a breakfast spot _____

33. an office supply store _____

34. an historic site _____

35. a golf course _____

36. a plant nursery _____

TARGET AREA 6: Word Retrieval   States and Cities

DIRECTIONS: Next to each city, write the name of its state.

EXAMPLE: Denver   *Colorado* _____

1. Wichita   _____

2. Boston   _____

3. Providence   _____

4. Pittsburgh   _____

5. Milwaukee   _____

6. Memphis   _____

7. San Diego   _____

8. Indianapolis   _____

9. Houston   _____

10. Palm Beach   _____

11. Cleveland _____

12. Baton Rouge _____

13. Lexington _____

14. Des Moines _____

15. St. Paul _____

16. New Orleans _____

17. Omaha _____

18. Portland _____

19. Salt Lake City _____

20. Green Bay _____

21. Detroit _____

22. Birmingham _____

23. Atlantic City _____

276

24. Savannah _____

25. Anchorage _____

26. Las Vegas _____

27. Phoenix _____

28. Boise _____

29. Baltimore _____

30. Santa Fe _____

31. St. Louis _____

32. Little Rock _____

33. Williamsburg _____

34. Seattle _____

35. Buffalo _____

36. Fargo _____

TARGET AREA 6: Word Retrieval   Well-Known Places

DIRECTIONS: Write the name of the location where you would find each of the items.

EXAMPLE: Mt. Fuji _____ *Japan* _____

Cape Cod _____ *Massachusetts* _____

1. Niagara Falls _____

2. The Everglades _____

3. Pearl Harbor _____

4. Taj Mahal _____

5. Jefferson Memorial _____

6. Mall of America _____

7. Empire State Building _____

8. Nova Scotia _____

9. Buenos Aires _____

10. Blarney Stone _____

11. Venice _____

12. The Pentagon _____

13. The Alps _____

14. Wailing Wall _____

15. Chile _____

16. Panama Canal _____

17. Moscow _____

18. Nile River _____

19. Maui _____

20. The Alamo _____

21. The Pyramids _____

22. Toronto _____

23. Times Square _____

24. The Vatican _____

25. Calcutta _____

26. Red Square _____

27. Cairo _____

28. Long Island _____

29. Smoky Mountains _____

30. Death Valley _____

31. Juneau _____

32. The Colosseum _____

33. Madrid _____

34. Jerusalem _____

35. The Smithsonian _____

36. Mt. Rushmore _____

37. Statue of Liberty _____

38. Fisherman's Wharf _____

39. Havana _____

40. Amsterdam _____

41. Grand Canyon _____

42. Mormon Tabernacle _____

43. The Rose Bowl _____

44. Liberty Bell _____

45. Martha's Vineyard _____

46. Eiffel Tower _____

47. Rocky Mountains _____

48. Kenya _____

TARGET AREA 6: Word Retrieval   Famous Persons

DIRECTIONS: Write the full name of a person who fits each description.

EXAMPLE: a king ___*King George*_____

1. a comedian _____

2. an actor _____

3. a fashion designer _____

4. a Disney character _____

5. someone from the Bible _____

6. a vice president _____

7. an artist _____

8. a movie star _____

9. a governor _____

10. a singer _____

11. a newscaster _____

12. a chef _____

13. a singing group _____

14. an Olympic medal winner _____

15. a famous animal's name _____

16. an explorer _____

17. a head of a country _____

18. a person with a TV show _____

19. a composer _____

20. a senator _____

21. a rock star _____

22. a children's character _____

23. a deceased celebrity _____

TARGET AREA 6: Word Retrieval   Categories

DIRECTIONS: *The three things in each group can all be considered part of the same category. Think of a word or two that describes what they all have in common. Write those words on the line.*

EXAMPLE: chairs, tables, sofas

These are ___*pieces of furniture*_____

1. bear, cow, groundhog

   These are _____

2. navy, yellow, pink

   These are _____

3. Ford, Lincoln, Clinton

   These are _____

4. trout, haddock, perch

   These are _____

5. Hershey, Godiva, Ghiradelli

   These are _____

6. Sears, Macy's, Target

   These are _____

7. crow, bluejay, robin

These are _____

8. melons, bananas, apples

These are _____

9. linen, silk, wool

These are _____

10. caller ID, call waiting, voicemail

These are _____

11. **Consumer Reports, Newsweek, Robb Report**

These are _____

12. rectangle, circle, square

These are _____

13. canoe, kayak, raft

These are _____

14. waltz, fox trot, cha-cha

These are _____

15. ape, chimpanzee, gorilla

These are _____

16. bag, canister, pocket

These are _____

17. CNN, MSNBC, C-Span

These are _____

18. Crock-Pot, wok, pressure cooker

These are _____

19. loafers, slippers, sandals

These are _____

20. Persian, Siamese, tabby

These are _____

21. granite, quartz, marble

These are _____

22. Nova Scotia, Quebec, Saskatchewan

These are _____

23. roulette, slots, blackjack

    These are _____

24. Monopoly, Scrabble, Trivial Pursuit

    These are _____

25. Oreos, Chips Ahoy, Mrs. Fields

    These are _____

26. buttons, zippers, snaps

    These are _____

27. fleece, quills, hide

    These are _____

28. lungs, appendix, liver

    These are _____

29. hoe, rake, spade

    These are _____

30. bell, whistle, siren

    These are _____

TARGET AREA 6: Word Retrieval   Occupations

DIRECTIONS: Write the correct answer after the question.

> EXAMPLE: If you wanted your portrait painted, who would you call?
>
> *an artist*

1. If your home were robbed, who would you call?

2. If you needed a flower arrangement, who would you call?

3. If a water pipe in your house burst, who would you call?

4. If your car wouldn't start, who would you call?

5. If you had questions about a prescription, who would you call?

6. If a dog needed medical attention, who would you take it to?

7. If you wanted advice on what cut of meat to buy, who would you ask?

   _____

8. If you wanted someone to take your order in a restaurant, who would you ask?

   _____

9. If you wanted to talk to the person in charge at a store, who would you ask to see?

   _____

10. If you wanted someone who would rid your home of bugs, who would you call?

    _____

11. If you wanted to know how much a ring you own is worth, who would you see?

    _____

12. If you wanted to buy into a mutual fund, who would you see?

    _____

13. If you wanted to get over a fear of heights, who would you see?

    _____

14. If you wanted to get your eyes checked, who would you see?

_____

15. If you wanted to get in better physical shape, who would you see?

_____

16. If you wanted someone to stay with a child while you were away, who would you hire?

_____

17. If you wanted someone else to cook the food for your party, who would you hire?

_____

18. If you wanted someone to cut and style your hair, who would you call?

_____

19. If you wanted to complain about your local taxes, who would you see?

_____

20. If you wanted to write a letter to a newspaper, who would you write it to?

_____

TARGET AREA 6: Word Retrieval   Descriptions

DIRECTIONS: Read the description. Write the name of what it describes on the line.

> EXAMPLE: It is an international sports competition that takes place
> every four years in the summer and in the winter.
> What is it?
>
> *the Olympic Games*

1. This is a national monument in New York Harbor. It is a figure of a lady holding a torch. What is it?

   _____

2. This is our national bird. It has a bald head and is pictured on a 50-cent piece. What is it?

   _____

3. This is a popular soft drink that contains carbonated water, sugar, caramel color, phosphoric acid, caffeine, and citric acid. What is it?

   _____

4. This is something that motorcycle drivers and riders wear on their heads for protection. What is it?

   _____

5. It is considered lucky to find one of these small plants. It is green and has a certain number of heart-shaped leaves. What is it?

_____

6. This is something that someone must have before they can legally operate a car. What is it?

_____

7. This is a brand of coffee that originated in Seattle. The brand has more than 10,000 coffee shops throughout the U.S. What is it?

_____

8. This is a part of the body that must keep beating in order for us to stay alive. What is it?

_____

9. Skiers use this to get from the bottom of a hill to the top. What is it?

_____

10. This is a vegetable that is green on the outside and white on the inside. It is used to make pickles. What is it?

_____

11. This is a list of topics in alphabetical order found at the end of some books. What is it?

_____

12. This is the place you put an electrical cord into a wall. What is it?

_____

13. This is what people look into when shaving or putting on makeup. What is it?

_____

14. This is the part of a computer that helps you move the cursor around the screen. What is it?

_____

15. This is a way to exercise your brain. You fill letters and words into a grid of black and white squares. You can find one in most newspapers. What is it?

_____

16. This is a vehicle that operates on a track underground. Each car can hold around 50 people. What is it?

_____

17. This is what you sleep in when you are camping. What is it?

_____

18. This is an indoor room where you can lift weights, or exercise with others. What is it?

_____

19. This is a type of vehicle which shovels snow from roads or driveways. What is it?

_____

20. This is an instrument used by a person talking to a large group so that his voice will be heard by everyone. What is it?

_____

21. This is the name of the piece of paper someone receives when they graduate from a school or special course. What is it?

_____

22. This is what several sentences grouped together with the same idea is called. What is it?

_____

23. This is the food we get from bees. What is it?

_____

24. These can develop in your teeth if you don't brush and floss on a regular basis. What are they called?

_____

25. These plants are found on beaches near saltwater. They are dark green or black and feel slimy. What are they called?

_____

26. These are things so small they can only be seen under a microscope. We keep our hands and food clean to avoid getting them in our bodies. What are they?

_____

27. This is an animal that looks for his shadow every February. If he sees his shadow, people say that there will be six more weeks of winter. What is it?

_____

28. This is kept between people. It is information shared with someone trusted that no one else knows. What is it called?

_____

29. This is something with sticky edges that you place over a wound to keep it clean. What is it?

_____

30. This type of boat carries cars and people over water from shore to shore. What is it?

_____

31. This is something people look for in oysters. It is small and hard and used in jewelry. What is it?

_____

TARGET AREA 6: Word Retrieval   Parts to Whole

DIRECTIONS: The three items listed on each line are all parts of a whole thing. Decide what whole the items are a part of, and write it on the line.

EXAMPLE: drumstick, breast, thigh

parts of a turkey

1. stage, seats, curtain

   _____

2. best man, rings, vows

   _____

3. expiration date, embossed numbers, your signature

   _____

4. tomato, ground beef, onion

   _____

5. sheet, blanket, mattress

   _____

6. sleeve, collar, buttons

   _____

7. flour, butter, eggs

_____

8. pages, table of contents, paper

_____

9. stalls, hay, troughs

_____

10. drawers, wood, knobs

_____

11. stems, buds, thorns

_____

12. nose, mouth, eyes

_____

13. laces, sole, heel

_____

14. icing, layers, batter

_____

15. carburetor, transmission, battery

_____

16. editorial, sports section, front page

_____

17. shell, yolk, white

_____

18. tinsel, strings of lights, ornaments

_____

19. feather, beak, claws

_____

20. sink, tub, toilet

_____

21. elbow, wrist, shoulders

_____

22. gutters, chimney, shingles

_____

TARGET AREA 6: Word Retrieval

Commonalities

DIRECTIONS: The two things listed in each item have something in common. Write what they have in common on the line.

> EXAMPLE: Rockies, Adirondacks *__mountains in the U.S.__*

1. Sea World, Cedar Point _____

2. Chanel No. 5, Windsong _____

3. Rolling Stones, Guns N' Roses _____

4. **Let's Make a Deal, Deal or No Deal** _____

5. Eukanuba, Purina _____

6. Catholic, Jewish _____

7. Diet Dr. Pepper, Pepsi-Lite _____

8. Crest, Colgate _____

9. Cheddar, Swiss _____

10. Wendy's, McDonald's _____

11. State Farm, Prudential _____

12. Redskins, Dolphins _____

13. Saturn, Jupiter _____

14. basil, oregano _____

15. Judge Judy, Rachael Ray _____

16. Schlitz, Budweiser _____

17. Nabisco, Keebler _____

18. Whirlpool, Hotpoint _____

19. Hertz, Avis _____

20. Vera Wang, Giorgio Armani _____

21. Mrs. Butterworth, Aunt Jemima _____

22. Bounty, Viva _____

23. Rice Chex, Raisin Bran _____

24. Lowe's, Home Depot _____

25. Yellowstone, Yosemite _____

26. butter pecan, chocolate chip _____

27. I-75, I-90 _____

28. CVS, Rite-Aid _____

29. over easy, scrambled _____

30. Delta, American _____

31. Nike, Adidas _____

32. arthritis, bursitis _____

33. Dentyne, Trident _____

34. Evian, Aquafina _____

35. Big Dipper, planets _____

TARGET AREA 6: Word Retrieval   Reason for Fame

DIRECTIONS: Explain in a few words why each person is famous.

EXAMPLE: Robin Williams	*he is a comedian and actor*

1. Houdini _____

2. Muhammed Ali _____

3. Tiger Woods _____

4. Paul McCartney _____

5. Michelle Obama _____

6. Michael Phelps _____

7. Shrek _____

8. William Shakespeare _____

9. Celine Dion _____

10. Arnold Schwarzenegger _____

11. Homer and Marge Simpson _____

12. Smokey the Bear _____

13. Joe Biden _____

14. Scarlett O'Hara _____

15. Leonardo da Vinci _____

16. Harry Potter _____

17. Oprah Winfrey _____

18. Al Gore _____

19. Helen Keller _____

20. Jodie Foster _____

21. Willy Wonka _____

22. Martin Luther King _____

23. Paul Revere _____

24. Tom Brokaw _____

25. Bill Gates _____

26. Hillary Clinton _____

27. Frankenstein _____

28. Henry Ford _____

29. Mary Poppins _____

30. Anderson Cooper _____

31. Kobe Bryant _____

32. Evel Knievel _____

33. Sarah Palin _____

34. Frank Lloyd Wright _____

35. Steven Spielberg _____

TARGET AREA 7:
Answer Key to Selected Exercises

TARGET AREA 7: Answer Key to Selected Exercises

This Answer Key provides answer options for most of the exercises. In some cases, the answers are open-ended and should be looked at individually and are not included in the key. Other answers could be varied and correct as long as they make sense. There may be a different interpretation or thought process behind an answer. There may be variations in word order or alternate answers. In a few exercises, one **possible** set of answers is given and is only listed to give you an idea of a sample answer. The answers in each exercise are shown as a group as indicated by the page numbers. An exercise will be marked as "answer will vary" if each answer should be looked at separately.

Pages 15 – 18

1. nail
2. fall
3. on
4. beer
5. blades
6. cereal
7. Tiffany's
8. reserve
9. cavities
10. battery
11. speech
12. hurricane
13. jokes
14. blinds
15. meringue
16. Republican
17. lipstick
18. paper
19. dinner
20. hits
21. freckles
22. racket
23. candy
24. magazine
25. art
26. handle

Pages 19 – 22

1. fight
2. smells
3. tiger
4. robins
5. blizzard
6. chilly
7. rent
8. peach

9. leopard
10. registered
11. withdrew
12. valuable
13. hard-boiled
14. zipper
15. bottle
16. candidate
17. boots
18. tunnel
19. smoke
20. groceries
21. gravel
22. spare
23. Labor
24. CEO
25. flashlight

Pages 23 – 27

1. wallet
2. tricycle
3. essential
4. Historical
5. flood
6. starvation
7. insulation
8. pastor
9. egotistical
10. football
11. contestant
12. subscription
13. ankle
14. stock
15. jacket
16. souvenirs
17. club
18. cemetery
19. height

20. fat
21. neutral
22. dehumidifier
23. smoke
24. sports
25. portrait
26. ruby
27. splinter
28. radio
29. mahogany
30. widow

Pages 28 – 31

1. Rushmore – mountain
   Mississippi – river
   Seattle – city
   Pacific – ocean
2. Einstein – scientist
   Boone – pioneer
   Geronimo – native American
   Edison – inventor
3. maple – sap
   oak – acorns
   evergreen – needles
   crabapple – blossoms
4. milk – homogenized
   cider – juice
   soft drink – carbonated
   champagne – alcoholic
5. Excedrin – aspirin
   Windex – cleaner
   Tide – detergent
   Mitchum – deodorant
6. Everglades – Florida
   Niagara Falls – New York
   Golden Gate Bridge – California
   Gettysburg – Pennsylvania
7. Ottawa – Canada
   London – England
   New Delhi – India
   Tokyo – Japan
8. Peter Pan – Captain Hook
   Prince Charming – Cinderella
   Red Riding Hood – Big Bad Wolf
   Hansel – Gretel
9. 60 Minutes – TV show
   Hamlet – play
   Star Wars – movie
   Alice in Wonderland – book
10. Maya Angelou – poet
    Pablo Picasso – artist
    Mark Twain – writer
    Frederic Chopin – composer

11. Jamaica – island
    Brazil – country
    Asia – continent
    Geneva – city
12. Ronald – Reagan
    George – Bush
    Barack – Obama
    Bill – Clinton
13. sticks – drum
    keys – piano
    bow – cello
    strings – harp
14. colt – horse
    kid – goat
    lamb – sheep
    calf – cow
15. seeds – pumpkin
    lead – pencil
    ink – pen
    blood – veins
16. Michael Jordan – basketball
    Hank Aaron – baseball
    Walter Payton – football
    Wayne Gretzky – hockey
17. hamburger – meatloaf
    noodles – lasagna
    dough – pizza
    eggs – omelet
18. Tony Bennett – singer
    Jeff Foxworthy – comedian
    Will Smith – actor
    Rudy Giuliani – politician

Pages 32 – 35

1. Restaurants, sit-down, menu, server, bill, tip
2. 8 arms, salt, eat, pets
3. Shakespeare, plays, Macbeth, England, 16th
4. Benjamin, library, Declaration, Independence, picture, hundred
5. President, White, U.S., Washington, D.C., Congress, Senate, Representatives
6. red, green, right, stop, traffic
7. Hummingbirds, smallest, long, nectar, wings, fly
8. Movies, G, age, X, adults, is not
9. Beavers, flat, buck, wood, swim, dams
10. Hawaii, state, islands, Pacific, Honolulu, pineapple
11. Pizza, tomato, cheese, baked, slice
12. Neil, astronaut, Apollo 11, the moon, first, walk
13. average, 7, dreams, remembers, 1/3, sleeping
14. organ, keys, keys, hands, pedals, feet

Pages 36 – 41

1. lag behind
2. fall down
3. meat
4. pull apart
5. look forward to
6. a medication
7. fabric
8. empty
9. dark syrup
10. hair
11. written information
12. health resort
13. disguise
14. picture
15. gently urge
16. good
17. relax
18. delay
19. ten years
20. end
21. drain
22. clear plastic
23. dog
24. around something
25. bomb
26. speaking
27. choice
28. finger joint

Pages 42 – 47

Answers may vary. Listen to individual explanations.
1. in an orchard, in a restaurant, at a roadside stand, from a vending machine
2. chalk, marker, pencil, crayon
3. credit card, paper clip, snapshot
4. cheese, cream
5. movies, books, shelves, maps
6. pillowcase, washcloth, quilt
7. aspirin, nap, warm drink
8. beans, cake, salad
9. magazines, gum, shampoo, shoelaces
10. headphones, pitcher, rags
11. sweater, wool jacket
12. teething ring, diapers, bib, stuffed animal
13. deeds, stocks, jewelry, wills
14. dirt, watering cans, seedlings, pots
15. facebook, eBay, Google
16. envelope, address, stamp
17. court, opponent, racket, net
18. toast, garter toss, tiered cake
19. past returns, receipts
20. safety glasses, wire, pliers, wrench, utility knife
21. chips and salsa, cheese and crackers, popcorn and pretzels
22. tent, matches, lantern

Pages 48 – 53

The words are listed in the order they should be put in the sentence.
1. car, ad, paper, cost
2. poker, TV, popcorn, beer
3. accident, intersection, police, ambulance
4. weather, board, rescheduled, 8:00
5. clerk, refund, price, merchandise
6. violence, movies, contributing, crime
7. flight, Miami, travel, Nassau
8. sirloin, steak, medium, well
9. Congress, tax, vetoed, session
10. hour, traffic, light, commuters
11. Government, statistics, Americans, cars
12. sleep, exercise, vitamins, healthy
13. Italian, lasagna, Mexican, tacos or Mexican, tacos first
14. morning, orchard, apples, applesauce
15. tuition, high, afford, pay
16. photographer, trouble, pose, pictures
17. cold, state, west, cooler, temperatures
18. President, State, Union, Address, Wednesday
19. Retrievers, Collies, pets, families, children
20. hates, cold, loves, heat, Florida
21. heard, plasma, cost, decided, expensive
22. trap, catch, raccoon, lives, deck
23. X-ray, fracture, bone, joint, finger
24. storm, power, schools, closed, stores, open OR storm, power, stores, open, schools, closed

Pages 57 – 62

1. beverage
2. game show
3. numbers
4. fall
5. water
6. Japan
7. apple
8. opera
9. neck
10. gas
11. cantaloupe
12. plains
13. higher
14. killed
15. drink

16. hot
17. jog
18. actor
19. feet
20. waitress
21. country
22. DVD
23. football
24. dance
25. horses
26. pedometer
27. leaves
28. dead
29. Thanksgiving
30. facets
31. rattlesnake
32. sponge
33. auditorium
34. Yahtzee
35. hands
36. microwave
37. jack-in-the-pulpit
38. tetanus
39. expressway
40. trowel

Pages 63 – 66

1. yes
2. no (electricity)
3. yes
4. no (kid)
5. yes
6. no (sucks food into mouth)
7. no (yoga is exercise)
8. no (jellybeans are candy)
9. no (gargle it)
10. no (too hard)
11. no (maybe lose cones)
12. yes
13. no (DVD)
14. yes
15. yes
16. no (it's a seashell)
17. no (366)
18. yes
19. no (goal)
20. yes
21. yes
22. yes
23. no (larger)
24. yes
25. yes
26. no (English prime minister)
27. no (air)
28. no (it's frozen)

29. no (koala is animal)
30. yes
31. no (heart)
32. no (flower bulbs)
33. yes
34. no (disease)
35. yes
36. no (over-the-counter)
37. no (story character)
38. no (New Orleans)
39. yes
40. no (wild west showman)
41. yes
42. no (steering wheel)
43. no (on your head)
44. yes
45. yes
46. no (not normally)
47. yes
48. no
49. yes

Pages 67 – 68

1. no (in your state)
2. probably not
3. no (after)
4. yes
5. yes (for most people)
6. yes
7. yes
8. yes
9. no (8th)
10. yes
11. yes
12. no (southeast)
13. no (woman)
14. no (too high)
15. yes
16. yes
17. no (extra sensory perception)
18. yes
19. no (bachelor's degree first)
20. no (PST-Pacific Standard Time)
21. no (corporation larger)
22. no (quarter pound = 4 ounces)
23. yes

Pages 69 – 72

1. T = True
2. F = False (warm regions)
3. T
4. T
5. F (Wales is a country)
6. F (Canadian has prime minister)

7. F (government program)
8. T
9. F (national court)
10. F (spice)
11. T
12. F (person)
13. T
14. F (money)
15. T
16. T
17. F (illegal drug)
18. F (two types of fuel)
19. F (brings money)
20. F (people held by others)
21. T
22. T
23. T
24. T
25. F (heart)
26. T
27. F (TV stations)
28. F (B is for bacon)
29. F (keys are pressed)
30. T
31. F (singer)
32. T
33. T
34. T
35. F (small mammal)
36. T
37. F (type of skate)
38. T
39. F (electronic mail)
40. T
41. T
42. T
43. F (stuffed bears)
44. T
45. T
46. F (Big Easy)
47. F (ice cream)

Pages 73 – 74

1. no (tooth trouble)
2. yes
3. no (furniture)
4. no (possible –usually meat or dairy)
5. yes
6. no
7. yes
8. yes
9. no (paper burns)
10. yes
11. no (numbers only)
12. no (by pair)

13. no (short ears, long neck)
14. yes
15. no (deaf)
16. yes
17. yes
18. no (Federal Express)
19. yes
20. no (cold)
21. yes
22. no (females)
23. yes

Pages 75 – 77

1. +
2. +
3. +
4. –
5. +
6. –
7. +
8. +
9. –
10. +
11. +
12. –
13. +
14. –
15. +
16. +
17. –
18. +
19. –
20. –
21. +
22. +
23. –
24. –
25. +
26. +
27. –
28. +
29. +
30. –
31. +
32. +
33. –
34. +
35. +
36. –

Pages 78 – 80

These answers are personal and should be looked at individually.

Pages 81 – 85

1. Kroger
2. crooked
3. five
4. hair
5. 300 feet
6. sit down
7. soap and water
8. excited
9. handsome thief
10. yelling
11. late pickup
12. turn right
13. started to rain
14. editor
15. six percent
16. 12
17. $649.95
18. Tuesday
19. three days in a row
20. strong, even
21. two
22. minimum daily requirements
23. Herman's Deli
24. standing ovation
25. protein diet
26. rings
27. $50 gift card
28. five-mile radius
29. many areas
30. JMJ Roofing
31. brownie
32. no

Pages 86 – 90

1. someone with no brothers or sisters
2. original idea
3. sale of things no longer needed
4. part of a baseball field
5. time-out during the day
6. place to keep money
7. way of sharing rides
8. with ice cream
9. someone whose kids have left home
10. used clothing
11. job through the night
12. show with real people / situations
13. place to buy tickets
14. distress from staying inside
15. someone who throws trash
16. someone who worries a lot
17. audition for actors
18. area of several connected stores
19. movie females will probably like

20. bathrooms
21. judge's order to not talk about a case
22. someone who saves a lot
23. woman who acts like a queen
24. promise for the future
25. people who take celebrity pictures
26. very, very close first and second place
27. continue regardless of obstacles

Pages 91 – 95

1. antifreeze
2. export
3. interview
4. exterior
5. disinfect
6. change
7. artificial
8. distant
9. rejected
10. herd
11. deflate
12. common
13. lovely
14. correct
15. supervisor
16. nervous
17. predict
18. arson
19. adoption
20. sandals
21. solitaire
22. cartoonist
23. fact
24. solar
25. exaggerate
26. croquet
27. award
28. roast
29. gulp
30. tarnish
31. illegible
32. corporation
33. imitate

Pages 96 – 99

1. yes
2. no
3. yes
4. no
5. yes
6. yes
7. yes
8. no

9. no
10. yes
11. no
12. no
13. yes
14. yes
15. yes
16. no
17. yes
18. no
19. no
20. yes
21. no
22. yes
23. no
24. no
25. no
26. no

Pages 100 – 104

1. S (same)
2. D (different)
3. D
4. D
5. S
6. S
7. S
8. S
9. D
10. S
11. S
12. D
13. D
14. D
15. S
16. D
17. D
18. D
19. S
20. D
21. S
22. D
23. S
24. D
25. S
26. D
27. S
28. D
29. D
30. S
31. D
32. D
33. D
34. D
35. S

36. D
37. D
38. S
39. D
40. S
41. D
42. S

Pages 105 – 107

Answers will vary. The sentences can be changed in a number of ways and still make sense.

Pages 108 – 114

1. the woman
2. the dog
3. no
4. spring
5. Tom Hanks
6. black
7. Jane
8. Bob
9. yes
10. a cat
11. Bob
12. no
13. no
14. took a nap
15. the Johnsons
16. Mary
17. paint
18. Carol
19. Mark
20. both
21. her house
22. 3
23. 1
24. John
25. 2
26. 2
27. John
28. lights out
29. 4
30. 11
31. Todd
32. stocks
33. leasing

Pages 115 – 123

1. simmer, after, five minutes
2. yes, slow count to five, six inches
3. pick up card, nine, diamond
4. no, three minutes, one pint

5. no, no, sales
6. no, sandpaper, no
7. foil, 425, soft when fork in it
8. left, no, yes
9. shaving cream, no, wash the spot
10. 60 percent, 50, 30 mph
11. left, 203, second
12. 2, before, 3
13. yes, on left with red shutters, 3
14. Pat Fipps, blue pen, Jack Dunsburg
15. 10:40, no, no
16. 1:00 to 4:00, half hour, Saturday
17. 4, no, two months
18. no, no, bandages
19. 8:00 – 10:00, Dog Obedience, Investments
20. onions, garlic, 1 pound
21. yes, rash, yes
22. 9 to 11, Dancing with the Stars, answers will vary
23. every other day, shot, one cup three times a day (3 cups)
24. cheese and croutons, Ranch dressing, sour cream and parmesan cheese
25. 7, glasses and silverware and tablecloths, no, yes
26. by 9:30, Alex and Dan, probably Dan

Pages 124 – 127

1 (aspirin), 3, 2
2 (rug cleaner), 3, 1
3 (shampoo), 2, 1
2 (salad dressing), 3, 1
1 (sweater), 3, 2
3 (stock), 1, 2
3 (doctor), 2, 1
2 (radio), 3, 1
1 (spaghetti), 3, 2
1 (gas station), 2, 3
3 (Kool-Aid), 2, 1
2 (wallpaper), 1 3
3 (brownies), 2, 1
3 (microwave), 2, 1

Pages 128 – 133

1. D, B, A, C
2. C, D, B, A
3. D, A, B, C
4. D, C, B, A
5. A, B, D, C
6. C, B, A, D
7. D, A, C, B
8. D, B, A, C
9. C, D, B, A
10. A, D, B, C
11. C, A, B, D

Pages 134 – 138

1. It's on the tip of my tongue.
2. Absence makes the heart …
3. Never put off until tomorrow…
4. Leave no stone unturned.
5. Hope for the best and …
6. Here today, gone tomorrow
7. You get what you pay for.
8. Too many cooks spoil the broth.
9. Don't cry over spilled milk.
10. Chip off the old block
11. Actions speak louder than words.
12. Haste makes waste.
13. Squeaky wheel gets the grease.
14. You can't judge a book…
15. You hit the nail on the head.
16. Amy let the cat out of the bag.
17. Drown your sorrows.
18. No pain, no gain.

Pages 139 – 141

1. rodent (not human)
2. dominoes (not related to computer)
3. pyramids (not religious)
4. midnight (not light color)
5. pirate (not tool)
6. salad (not dessert)
7. chains (not money-related)
8. wallpaper (not for floors)
9. Den (not branch of government)
10. keys (not types of narcotics)
11. submarine (not space program)
12. SpongeBob (not superhero)
13. drums (not noise)
14. ASAP (not a product)
15. dime (not law-breaking term)
16. alibi (not food)
17. Friends (not movie)
18. stairs (not related to news)
19. briefly (not insect)
20. howdy (not good-bye in foreign)
21. foul (not related to labor)
22. accident (not banking term)
23. heater (not form of light)
24. au gratin (not egg dish)
25. party (not type of rest)
26. button (not strands of fiber)
27. closet (not carrying case)
28. markup (not low price)
29. aunt (not male)
30. cider (not carbonated)

Pages 145 – 148

1. listen
2. onion
3. picture
4. motor
5. earning
6. speak
7. healthy
8. business
9. sincere
10. journal
11. politics
12. normal
13. awards
14. unlimited
15. rooster
16. organize
17. package
18. leather
19. alarm
20. bureau
21. fabric
22. mineral
23. performance
24. figure
25. program
26. silence
27. kidnap
28. manicure
29. frail
30. absorb
31. identical
32. valuable
33. jealous
34. kitchen
35. mattress
36. conquer
37. wrestling
38. dependable
39. recognize
40. diplomatic
41. ointment

Pages 149 – 152

1. facility - 3
2. champagne - 2
3. crocodile - 3
4. dictionary - 2
5. vinyl - 1
6. accompany - 3
7. absolutely - 1
8. skiing - 2
9. beautiful - 3
10. surprise - 3
11. governor - 1
12. committee - 3
13. mayonnaise - 2
14. vanilla - 2
15. luncheon - 2
16. pumpkin - 1
17. secretary - 3
18. maximum - 2
19. eccentric - 2
20. raccoon - 2
21. ordinary - 1
22. nuisance - 2
23. fascinating - 1
24. cedar - 2
25. mechanic - 3
26. memorial - 2
27. guarantee - 1
28. pleasure - 3
29. manipulate - 1
30. territory – 2
31. occasion - 2
32. rhythm - 3
33. November - 1
34. February - 2
35. miniature - 3
36. volunteer - 1
37. shoulders - 3
38. rehearsal - 1
39. adequate - 2
40. physician - 2
41. abbreviation – 3

Pages 153 – 156

1. coopon - 2
2. hungery - 2
3. referance - 2
4. lodgical - 3
5. anounce - 3
6. dignosis - 1
7. watermellon - 2
8. laringitis - 2
9. endevear - 3
10. probabely - 2
11. spinatch - 2
12. bicicle - 1
13. groutchy - 2
14. razsberry - 3
15. innosent - 1
16. natuerally - 2
17. gardner - 3
18. umanimous - 1
19. karesene - 2
20. trajedy - 3
21. jellousy - 1
22. medisine - 2

23. valueble - 1
24. frushtrated - 3
25. orijinal - 2
26. holliday - 2
27. negoshiate - 1
28. weapen - 2
29. sckedule - 3
30. ellevater - 1
31. chockolate - 3
32. reasonble - 1
33. laufhter - 2
34. generus - 3
35. mashine - 2
36. toester - 3
37. delishious – 1
38. brillant – 3
39. nomminate – 2
40. opinon – 1
41. yoreself - 2

Pages 157 – 159

The answers are reading across.
1. short, chair, chest, there, chart, then, thirsty, shade
2. meet, squeeze, believe, being, piece, weight, ceiling, friend
3. contain, beauty, insult, condemn, continue, index, before, belief
4. extra, unite, exact, excuse, percent, perhaps, unhappy, perform
5. common, transport, internal, transfer, translate, complex, interview, company
6. goat, broom, deep, street, need, toast, mood, load
7. night, phony, whale, photo, phrase, why, high, whip
8. lettuce, middle, willow, battle, puddle, butter, collar, hidden
9. flag, plug, blend, floor, please, flimsy, plead, blast
10. string, scratch, strong, shrill, script, strain, scrape, shriek
11. noise, guilty, stairs, choice, train, daisy, quick, squirrel
12. decided, suite, evidence, waiter, voices, spider, license, video
13. document, witness, cement, vacation, business, element, question, witness
14. tennis, success, different, offered, accept, coffee, kennel, soccer

Pages 160 – 162

Answers will vary. If a word is formed using the letters given, it is correct.

Pages 163 – 165

1. beg, bug, big, bag
2. pet, Pat, pit, pot
3. mist, mast, most, must
4. Dick, duck, deck, dock
5. pin, pen, pun, pan
6. hen, Ben, Ken or Len, men, ten
7. rush, bush, hush, push
8. Ray or Jay, hay, May, pay
9. dill, pill, hill, bill
10. cold, told, gold, sold
11. rest, nest, vest, best

Pages 166 – 168

1. seed, peek, heel, beef
2. hair, main, fail, said
3. hour, loud, noun, soup
4. loaf, toad, soak, foam
5. duet, Tues, fuel, sued
6. weak, pear, veal, deaf
7. lied, view, diet, pier
8. sure, June, cube, nude
9. race, tame, wave, page
10. joke, vote, mole, bone
11. rice, time, wife, five

Pages 169 – 170

<u>Sample</u> answers are given. There may be other words that can be formed so check each word individually.
1. glass
2. berry
3. gallon
4. leave
5. poor
6. kind
7. anchor
8. seven
9. horse
10. judge
11. easy
12. habit
13. puzzle
14. plastic
15. brown
16. knob
17. organ
18. radio
19. match
20. thorn
21. pyramid
22. image
23. light
24. shared

25. rodeo
26. person
27. strong
28. banana
29. after
30. camp
31. drain
32. whale
33. blood
34. ground
35. cute
36. closet
37. alike
38. object
39. world
40. concert
41. piano
42. liquid
43. task
44. sausage

Pages 171 – 172

1. difficult
2. earthquake
3. magician
4. millionaire or billionaire or zillionaire
5. elephant
6. candidate
7. industry
8. screwdriver
9. jealous
10. buffalo
11. celery
12. apartment
13. telephone
14. accept
15. pumpkin or bumpkin
16. finger
17. ambulance
18. thousand
19. decision or derision
20. beginning
21. available
22. rattlesnake
23. scrapbook
24. appointment
25. basketball
26. grapefruit
27. cancellation
28. animal
29. cushion
30. umbrella
31. illustrate
32. vertical
33. successful

34. arrow or allow or aglow
35. alphabet
36. happiness
37. photograph
38. binoculars
39. telescope
40. original
41. mountain
42. because
43. sympathy
44. knowledge

Pages 173 – 174

One set of <u>sample</u> answers is given. There are other words that can be formed so check each word individually.

1. peak
2. dive
3. tool
4. hose
5. coat
6. have
7. best
8. cool
9. fix
10. wash
11. bird
12. soak
13. heel
14. grab
15. ring
16. wait
17. year
18. blue
19. thaw
20. lion
21. hits
22. foam
23. port
24. warm
25. less
26. wing
27. soup
28. flame
29. book
30. pint
31. chest
32. patch
33. yell
34. chip
35. scold
36. boss
37. take
38. stay
39. weed

40. chose
41. just
42. tube
43. shore
44. wrap

Pages 175 – 176

One set of <u>sample</u> answers is given. There are other words that can be formed so check each one individually.

1. relish
2. corner
3. mistake
4. polite
5. repeat
6. gallery
7. electric
8. sandy
9. prepare
10. subject
11. column
12. passion
13. stamp
14. bleed
15. shrug
16. couple
17. blouse
18. chute
19. dessert
20. swimming
21. scratch
22. allow
23. germs
24. living
25. initial
26. overrule
27. banner
28. quiz
29. railing
30. frown
31. squish
32. chilled
33. jockey
34. language
35. keeper
36. examine
37. travel
38. handsome
39. nonfiction
40. tackle
41. exchange
42. progress
43. grease
44. location

Pages 177 – 178

One set of <u>sample</u> answers is given. There are many other words that can be formed.

1. terrible
2. florists
3. mustard
4. lobby
5. travel
6. burping
7. brass
8. juice
9. blender
10. curious
11. alive
12. cheek
13. balance
14. pebbles
15. whistle
16. awake
17. March
18. fresh
19. sheriff
20. clown
21. wall
22. buddy
23. strip
24. major
25. house
26. faint
27. spaces
28. purple
29. choose
30. thick
31. stuff
32. village
33. lawyer
34. seaweed
35. leave
36. cracker
37. supplies
38. leash
39. silver
40. adult
41. yearly
42. sesame
43. answer
44. fourth

Pages 179 – 181

1. bear
2. nose
3. wear
4. hear
5. grown

6. doe
7. sell
8. towed
9. wore
10. rose
11. heal
12. main
13. pear
14. guessed
15. Their
16. flu
17. due
18. raise
19. through
20. cereal
21. stare
22. need
23. wait
24. sent
25. fur
26. meet
27. course
28. shoot
29. peace
30. brakes
31. won, prize
32. blew, hair

Pages 182 – 184

One set of _sample_ answers is given. There are many other words that can be formed.

1. bedroom
2. together
3. spoon
4. tribe
5. desk
6. sale
7. roar
8. string
9. decide
10. session
11. Chicago
12. wouldn't
13. zero
14. need, knead
15. success
16. international (13 letters)
17. to, us
18. finger
19. example
20. quiet
21. throw
22. practical (9 letters)
23. swimmer
24. airplane

25. dribble
26. child / children
27. lunch
28. proof

Pages 187 – 190

Answer may vary. One set of _possible_ answers is given.

1. trash
2. receptionist
3. party
4. receipt
5. club soda
6. dry cleaners
7. emergency center
8. Tree trimmers
9. Jogging
10. tied
11. strawberry
12. saw
13. Bowling
14. cheese
15. blood
16. haircut
17. knit
18. liberal
19. chicken
20. shot
21. coffee table
22. forehead
23. zip
24. partner
25. paroled
26. applauded
27. cancer
28. staircase
29. defroster
30. trigger
31. drawer
32. hydrant
33. directions
34. train

Pages 191 – 193

One set of _sample_ answers is given. There are many other words or phrases that can be formed.

1. sky
2. potatoes
3. flake
4. over
5. Tower
6. Erie
7. Island
8. lash

9. Pole
10. ball
11. England
12. pudding
13. tea
14. vision
15. cube
16. blister
17. card
18. payment
19. pepper
20. underwear
21. States
22. throw
23. glasses
24. broken
25. age
26. news
27. sauce
28. bulb
29. light
30. straw
31. conditioner
32. me-downs
33. proof
34. utilities
35. decker
36. class

Pages 194 – 197

Answers may vary. One set of <u>possible</u> answers is given.
1. golf, Friday
2. speaker, clap
3. waitress, sundaes
4. amazed, price
5. Arizona, climate
6. locked, left
7. smartest, met
8. tired, sleep
9. chicken breasts, vegetables
10. Hockey, sport
11. spelling, reception
12. kitten, couch
13. cracker, cardboard
14. blueberry, glazed
15. grease, arm
16. wife, lodge
17. teenager, sleeping
18. fur, soft
19. drink, driving
20. mowed, water
21. waiter, tray
22. twins, six
23. laughed, joke

24. pizza, cake
25. gym, pounds
26. Newspapers, lawn
27. soup, pepper
28. vitamins, coffee

Pages 198 – 212

Answers will vary. Check each sentence individually to see if it makes sense.

Pages 215 – 219

No answers are provided. Each sentence will read the same except for the one or two new word that are substituted.

Pages 220 – 224

Answers will vary. Each new sentence will include one or two words from the other sentences to form one precise sentence.

Pages 225 – 228

1. Colonel Smith works in the first building on the boulevard.
2. The address is 430 Oak Avenue, Saint Louis, Missouri.
3. Your next appointment is on Tuesday, November third at two-thirty.
4. Maple Road is two miles on your right.
5. The package weighed forty-seven pounds, three and a half ounces.
6. Mister William Day Junior is an attorney.
7. Eggs cost two dollars, eighty-nine cents a dozen and milk costs two dollars thirty-nine cents a half gallon.
8. Three feet equals one yard.
9. He received a bachelor of science from Michigan State University.
10. The manager hired an assistant on Monday.
11. The temperature is seventy-two degrees Fahrenheit in New York City.
12. It is four months until Christmas.
13. Los Angeles is the second largest city in the United States of America.
14. The apartment has fifteen hundred square feet, dining room, and a fireplace.
15. Doctor Kelly of the Federal Bureau of Investigation called General Hicks of the Central Intelligence Agency.
16. The recipe called for two cups and three teaspoons of sugar.
17. My sports utility vehicle gets about thirty miles per gallon when traveling at fifty-five miles per hour.

18. Sales tax in Florida is six percent.
19. Connecticut is northeast of Texas.
20. Professor Snyder is head of the government department.
21. The order was a bacon, lettuce, and tomato on rye, a Doctor Pepper, and French fries.
22. The emergency center is near the railroad crossing on Highway sixty-two.

Pages 229 – 232

Answers will vary. Each answer sentence should include all three words and make sense.

Pages 233 – 236

Answers will vary. Each answer sentence should make sense and, minimally, substitute the underlined words for another group of words.

Pages 237 – 240

Answers will vary. Each written sentence should make sense as an adequate answer for the question.

Pages 241 – 245

Answers will vary. Each written Q (question) should be a complete question that makes sense with the answer.

Pages 246 – 250

Answers will vary. Each written answer should be complete and answer the question.

Pages 251 – 255

Answers will vary. One set of possible answers is provided.
1. Suddenly the music stopped.
2. He found a chair and sat down.
3. She put on an old dress and left.
4. She picked flowers for the bouquet.
5. The directions were hard to understand.
6. The supervisor talked with the workers.
7. A law says you can't throw trash on highways.
8. It started as small disagreement but it got heated.
9. He walked fast because it was cold.
10. Our trip lasted four days longer than we thought it would.
11. I thought he had finished.
12. He noticed how pretty she was.
13. They have fence around their house so no one can see in or get in.
14. The constant noise gives me a headache.

15. The mouthy kid was told off.
16. The huge building was built very fast with poor quality.
17. The famous star talked about he is going to jail.
18. There were plenty of great appetizers.
19. Don't bother applying because we aren't hiring.
20. He was very angry about the little mistake.
21. The caring nurse tried to make the upset patient feel better.
22. The bottle fell and broke on the cement.
23. He was amazed I could come up with such a good idea.
24. She looks really out of place.
25. The game was called because of bad weather.
26. They are waiting to the last minute to decide if the quarterback will play.
27. It is warm but we get a lot of rain in the spring.

Pages 259 – 261

red: stop, cardinal, blood
yellow: corn, lemon, sun
blue: sky
green: grass, peas

New Orleans: Bourbon St., Mardi Gras
Hollywood: movie star, MGM, Rodeo Dr.
Alaska: Mt. McKinley, snow
Hawaii: pineapple, luau

John: Hancock, McCain, Travolta
Joe: Montana, Biden
Jack: Nicholson, Sprat
James: Brown, Bond

vegetable: artichoke, sprouts, yam
fruit: mango, fig
meat: knackwurst, veal
cheese: muenster, parmesan

Easter: bunny, colored egg
Christmas: wreath, Santa
4th of July: fireworks, picnic
Halloween: pumpkin, trick-or-treat, ghost

movie: **Titanic**, **Lion King**
cartoon: Bullwinkle, Bugs Bunny
comics: Ziggy, Peanuts
fairy tale: Cinderella, Red Riding Hood, Snow White

fur: skunk, cat, squirrel
hair: wig, toddler
feathers: woodpecker, peacock
scales: trout, goldfish

movie: **Casablanca**, **Jaws**
song: **Amazing Grace**, **Blue Moon**

TV show: **Meet the Press, Sesame Street, Good Morning America**
play: **Macbeth**

author: Charles Dickens, Danielle Steel
musician: Andrea Bocelli, Harry Connick Jr.
actor: George Clooney, Kate Winslet
politician: Nancy Pelosi, Barack Obama

Pages 262 – 264

These answers all depend on the personal information of the person writing the answers.

Pages 265 – 267

Answers will vary. They may be general or specific to the person.

Pages 268 – 270

Answers will vary as there are several possible brand names for each answer. One set of <u>possible</u> answers is shown.

1. Crest
2. Ben & Jerry
3. Bass
4. Starbucks
5. Miller
6. Kraft
7. Lean Cuisine
8. Progresso
9. Kellogg's
10. Kibbles & Bits
11. Parkay
12. Pepsi
13. Snickers
14. Samsung
15. Scrabble
16. Newsweek
17. Canon
18. Aleve
19. Pantene
20. New York Times
21. Whirlpool
22. Mobil
23. Buick
24. Arrid
25. Dove
26. Reebok
27. Charmin
28. Yoplait
29. Mrs. Smith
30. American Tourister
31. Little Caesar's
32. Stearns & Foster

33. Craftsman
34. Sylvania
35. Dell
36. Lenox

Pages 271 – 273

Answers will vary and depend on the personal preferences and location of the person writing the answers.

Pages 274 – 276

1. Kansas
2. Massachusetts
3. Rhode Island
4. Pennsylvania
5. Wisconsin
6. Tennessee
7. California
8. Indiana
9. Texas
10. Florida
11. Ohio
12. Louisiana
13. Kentucky
14. Iowa
15. Minnesota
16. Louisiana
17. Nebraska
18. Oregon
19. Utah
20. Wisconsin
21. Michigan
22. Alabama (or Michigan)
23. New Jersey
24. Georgia
25. Alaska
26. Nevada
27. Arizona
28. Idaho
29. Maryland
30. New Mexico
31. Missouri
32. Arkansas
33. Virginia
34. Washington
35. New York
36. North Dakota

Pages 277 – 280

Answers can be more specific and could vary. One set of very general answers is given.
1. New York / Canadian border
2. Florida

3. in Pacific Ocean
4. India
5. Washington, D.C.
6. Minnesota
7. New York – New York City
8. Canada
9. Argentina
10. Ireland
11. Italy
12. Washington D.C.
13. Europe – Switzerland
14. Middle East – Jerusalem
15. South America
16. Central America – Panama
17. Russia
18. Africa
19. Hawaii
20. San Antonio, Texas
21. Egypt
22. Ontario, Canada
23. New York – New York City
24. Italy
25. India
26. Moscow, Russia
27. Egypt
28. New York – New York City
29. southeastern states
30. California
31. Alaska
32. Greece
33. Spain
34. middle east
35. Washington D.C.
36. Washington
37. New York – New York City
38. California – San Francisco
39. Cuba
40. Netherlands
41. Arizona
42. Utah
43. California – Pasadena
44. Pennsylvania – Philadelphia
45. Massachusetts – Cape Cod
46. France – Paris
47. western states
48. Africa

Pages 281 – 282

Answers will vary. Check each one individually.

Pages 283 – 286

Answers can vary. One set of possible answers
is given.
1. animals

2. colors
3. former presidents
4. fish
5. chocolate brands
6. department stores
7. birds
8. fruit
9. fabrics
10. phone options
11. news magazines
12. shapes
13. small boats without motors
14. ballroom dances
15. related to monkeys
16. containers
17. cable news channels
18. cooking vessels
19. shoes
20. cats
21. rocks / minerals
22. Canadian provinces
23. casino games
24. board games
25. cookies
26. clothing fasteners
27. coverings on mammals
28. internal organs
29. garden tools
30. noises using object

Pages 287 – 289

Answers may vary. One set of <u>possible</u> answers
are given.
1. police
2. florist
3. plumber
4. AAA
5. pharmacist
6. veterinarian
7. butcher
8. waitress / waiter
9. manager
10. exterminator
11. jewelry appraiser
12. financial advisor / stock broker
13. psychologist
14. ophthalmologist
15. fitness trainer
16. sitter
17. caterer
18. stylist, barber
19. tax assessor or city manager
20. editor

Pages 290 – 294

1. Statue of Liberty
2. eagle
3. Coke or Pepsi
4. helmet
5. four-leaf clover
6. license
7. Starbucks
8. heart
9. chairlift or tow rope
10. cucumber
11. index
12. plug or outlet
13. mirror
14. mouse
15. crossword puzzle
16. subway
17. tent, RV
18. gym
19. plow
20. microphone or megaphone
21. diploma
22. paragraph
23. honey
24. cavities
25. seaweed or algae
26. germs or bacteria
27. groundhog
28. secret
29. bandage
30. ferry
31. pearl

Pages 295 – 297

Answers may vary. One set of possible answers is given.

1. theater
2. wedding
3. credit card
4. meatloaf or spaghetti sauce
5. bed
6. shirt or blouse
7. bread, cookie, or cake batter
8. magazine or book
9. stable
10. dresser or desk
11. roses
12. face
13. shoe
14. cake
15. car
16. newspaper
17. egg
18. Christmas tree

19. bird
20. bathroom
21. arm
22. roof

Pages 298 – 300

Answers may vary. One set of possible answers is given.

1. amusement parks
2. perfume
3. rock bands
4. game shows
5. dog food
6. religions
7. low-calorie soda pop
8. toothpaste
9. cheese
10. fast food places
11. insurance companies
12. football teams
13. planets
14. herbs
15. TV personalities
16. beer
17. crackers
18. appliance brands
19. car rental companies
20. fashion designers
21. food brands
22. paper towels
23. cereals
24. home improvement stores
25. national parks
26. ice cream flavors
27. interstate highways
28. drugstore chains
29. ways to cook eggs
30. airline companies
31. athletic shoe brands
32. painful joint conditions
33. chewing gum
34. bottled water
35. things seen in night sky

Pages 301 – 303

Answers may vary. General answers are given.

1. magician and escape artist
2. boxer
3. golfer
4. member of the Beatles, singer
5. wife of President Obama
6. Olympic gold-medal swimmer
7. giant ogre movie character
8. English playwright

9. singer
10. weightlifter, governor of California
11. animated couple with TV show
12. symbolic forest ranger bear
13. vice president under Barack Obama
14. female lead in **Gone with the Wind**
15. Italian artist and inventor
16. fictional character from book and movie series
17. successful entrepreneur and talk show host
18. vice president for Bill Clinton and environmentalist
19. an inspirational deaf and mute woman
20. actor and movie director
21. character who owns a chocolate factory
22. leader of the Civil Rights movement
23. colonial statesman who warned of a British invasion
24. former NBC reporter, anchor and commentator
25. founder and head of Microsoft Corp.
26. wife of President Bill Clinton who ran for president in 2008
27. monster of movie and book fame
28. developed Model T and founder of Ford Motor Co.
29. fictional nanny in movie
30. reporter and commentator
31. Basketball star
32. motorcycle daredevil
33. Alaska governor, ran for vice president with John McCain in 2008
34. architect with a distinct style
35. director / producer of major films